Praise for *Bodybuilding*

"If you're a fan of the sport, a bodybuilder yourself, or a coach, this book is for you. Arnold published his encyclopedia of bodybuilding back in 1995, and 23 years later we finally have an evidence-based, scientifically sound, upgraded text to progress the bodybuilding world forward. Excellent work, Cliff and Peter!"

Christopher Barakat, MS, ATC, CISSN
Coach, Educator, and Athlete

"With a bodybuilding guidebook written by Peter and Cliff, you are getting the input of an academic who specifically researches bodybuilding, and a coach who has seen it all and knows what works from years in the trenches. Additionally, both authors have experienced the stage as competitors and can communicate what it's like and what skills you need to succeed. This book has it all, both practical solutions and evidence-based guidelines. I couldn't recommend it more highly!"

Eric Helms, PhD, CSCS
Coach at 3D Muscle Journey, PNBA Pro Qualified Bodybuilder, and IPF Raw Powerlifter

"Science based with real-world experience, Cliff Wilson makes contest preparation easy to follow and understand. The bottom line is he gets results."

Donovan Strong
Strong Physiques, IFBB Pro Classic Physique, PNBA Pro Bodybuilder, and Lifetime Natural Competitor

"I've worked with Cliff for almost three years now, and he has literally changed my life. I came to him at a very unhealthy place, physically and mentally, but he has completely transformed me in all aspects of my athletic career and my life."

Chelsea Kamody
Science Teacher, Physics Professor, and Natural Bikini Competitor

"Unparalleled in its depth and breadth, this is the handbook that expert and novice bodybuilding coaches and competitors have all been waiting for."

Acadia Webber, MS
Nutrition and Training Coach at AcadiaFit LLC and PhD Student at University of South Florida

"Cliff Wilson is the best contest prep coach in the game, period. If you are interested in learning the most optimal ways to prepare your mind and body for the stage, then look no further. This book should be your bible if you have any motivation at all in being the best athlete you can be."

Gary Amlinger
WNBF Pro Natural Bodybuilder, WNBF World Championship Qualified Athlete, and Physique Coach

"Cliff and Peter have done an amazing job combining science with practicality to help both beginners and veterans better approach their contest preps."

Andrew Pardue, BS, CSCS, CISSN
Owner of APFitness LLC

"Industry experts Peter Fitschen and Cliff Wilson have joined forces to create the ultimate educational resource for any competitor, coach, or fitness enthusiast who wants to learn more about the process of competitive bodybuilding."

Allison Fahrenbach, BS, CPT, CSCC, CSN
Nutritionist and Physique Specialist, Owner of AFS Gym, and IPE Figure Pro Natural Athlete

"Prior to working with Cliff, I was taught that during contest prep you can only eat chicken breast or tilapia with broccoli or asparagus. Cliff has taught me how to count macros and use a variety of foods to meet my needs during prep. Variety is the spice of life, even during prep . . . who knew?"

Candice Scott
IFBB Pro Women's Physique

"In this book, as with Cliff's coaching, he leaves no stone unturned and provides a comprehensive guide to competing that you won't find anywhere else. I highly recommend picking up this guide before you start your next prep, whether it's your first or fifteenth bodybuilding contest prep."

Chris Elkins
WNBF Pro Natural Bodybuilder, Flexible Dieter, and Online Coach

"I have been a competitive bodybuilder for over 25 years, and this is the first book that truly covers every aspect of the sport of bodybuilding and fitness: how the sport began and its history, every federation (drug tested and nontested) and each division within the federations, the evolution of the male and female physiques throughout the years, and training and nutrition. I was particularly impressed with the detail in covering competition preparation and how gender, ethnicity, and a person's history with weight loss and body fat all factor into how you can tailor a meal plan to optimize their chances of a successful physique transformation. This book also addresses the old-school traditions and myths, as well as present-day practices, and it references current research to show what is true and accurate versus what is now obsolete. This is a must-have for any and all fitness athletes."

Philip M. Ricardo Jr.
Retired Marine and Multiple World Champion
Pro Natural Bodybuilder

"*Bodybuilding: The Complete Contest Preparation Handbook* is carefully researched, clearly written, and extremely thorough. Peter and Cliff have created an invaluable resource for anyone with an interest in bodybuilding. This book should be required reading for everyone who wants to compete!"

Jeff Nipard
Pro Natural Bodybuilder and Owner of Canada's
Most Subscribed Fitness YouTube Channel

"If you are looking for the most comprehensive guide to contest prep with the numerous factors to consider before, during, and after your bodybuilding season, this book is a must-read. These same principles were applied to my contest prep experience with Cliff Wilson as my coach—leading me to the 2017 WNBF Overall World Figure Championship. Cliff and Peter are two of the most talented coaching minds in the bodybuilding world today."

Katie Anne Rutherford
Owner of Power Fit Performance, WNBF and OCB World
Figure Champion, and Elite Natural Powerlifter

"If you want to win your next show, you gotta work with Team Wilson."

Mike Neumann
Owner of Fit Body U

"If you want a thorough guide to getting onstage, start here. Based on science and impeccably organized, this book will walk you through everything you need to know to optimize your physique leading up to a show—and how to get even better after it's done."

Brian Whitacre
2015 WNBF Worlds, 2015 IFPA Yorton Cup,
Overall Pro World Champion

"Few people find their true purpose in life, but when you find those who have, it's something else to watch happen. The amount of passion Cliff radiates is something you hardly ever see, and because of this he has been able to climb the ranks to world-class contest prep specialist. Most contest prep coaches who start to gain notoriety eventually end up a bit blinded by their own ego, but in Cliff's situation he has remained just as hungry as day one. When he dispenses information, you know it's because he has truly arrived at this conclusion and not because it fits his flavor of the week. Cliff is self-correcting in his approach; how many world-class standouts he has coached, and pushed to new levels, is evidence that his systems work. I would certainly recommend any physique coach take a moment to learn from a man who has exponentially surpassed what anyone would classify as a successful contest prep coach resume."

Alberto Nunez
WNBF Pro Natural Bodybuilder and Contest Prep Coach

"From the proper mind-set to your peaking strategy, this book has you covered. If you are serious about bringing your best to the stage, you do not want to miss this!"

Mikey Weiss
PNBA Pro Physique Natural Athlete
and DFAC Pro Natural Bodybuilder

"If you want the most thorough guide to contest prep available, this is it. It covers everything—not just the big stuff like dieting, but even details like choosing a sanction or choosing a division to compete in."

James Krieger, MS
Founder of Weightology LLC

(Continued at the end of the book)

BODYBUILDING

THE COMPLETE CONTEST PREPARATION HANDBOOK

PETER J. FITSCHEN, PHD, CSCS
FITBODY AND PHYSIQUE LLC

CLIFF WILSON
TEAM WILSON BODYBUILDING

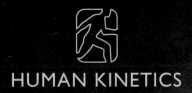

HUMAN KINETICS

Library of Congress Cataloging-in-Publication Data

Names: Fitschen, Peter J., 1986- author. | Wilson, Cliff, 1984- author.
Title: Bodybuilding : the complete contest preparation handbook / Peter J.
  Fitschen, PhD, CSCS., Cliff Wilson.
Description: Champaign, IL : Human Kinetics, [2020] | Includes
  bibliographical references and index.
Identifiers: LCCN 2018045409 (print) | LCCN 2018050257 (ebook) | ISBN
  9781492587491 (epub) | ISBN 9781492571346 (PDF) | ISBN 9781492571339
  (print)
Subjects: LCSH: Bodybuilding--Training. | Bodybuilding--Competitions. |
  Bodybuilders--Nutrition.
Classification: LCC GV546.5 (ebook) | LCC GV546.5 .F57 2020 (print) | DDC
  796.41--dc23
LC record available at https://lccn.loc.gov/2018045409

ISBN: 978-1-4925-7133-9 (print)

This publication is written and published to provide accurate and authoritative information relevant to the subject matter presented. It is published and sold with the understanding that the author and publisher are not engaged in rendering legal, medical, or other professional services by reason of their authorship or publication of this work. If medical or other expert assistance is required, the services of a competent professional person should be sought.

The web addresses cited in this text were current as of October 2018, unless otherwise noted.

Senior Acquisitions Editor: Roger W. Earle; **Managing Editor:** Karla Walsh; **Copyeditor:** Michelle Horn; **Proofreader:** Leigh Keylock; **Indexer:** Dan Connolly; **Permissions Manager:** Martha Gullo; **Graphic Designer:** Sean Roosevelt; **Cover Designer:** Keri Evans; **Cover Design Associate:** Susan Rothermel Allen; **Photographs (front cover):** Courtesy of Anna McManamey and Sam Okunola; **Photographs (back cover):** Courtesy of Doug Miller, Cyd Gillon, Valentine Ezugha, and Nadine Schmidt; **Photo Asset Manager:** Laura Fitch; **Photo Production Manager:** Jason Allen; **Senior Art Manager:** Kelly Hendren; **Illustrations:** © Human Kinetics; **Printer:** Walsworth

Printed in the United States of America   10 9 8 7 6 5 4 3

The paper in this book was manufactured using responsible forestry methods.

Human Kinetics
1607 N. Market Street
Champaign, IL 61820
USA

United States and International
Website: **US.HumanKinetics.com**
Email: info@hkusa.com
Phone: 1-800-747-4457

Canada
Website: **Canada.HumanKinetics.com**
Email: info@hkcanada.com

For information about Human Kinetics' coverage in other areas of the world, please visit our website: **www.HumanKinetics.com**

E7401

Tell us what you think!
Human Kinetics would love to hear what we can do to improve the customer experience. Use this QR code to take our brief survey.

BODYBUILDING

THE COMPLETE CONTEST PREPARATION HANDBOOK

CONTENTS

Foreword x • Preface xi • Acknowledgments xii • Photo Credits xiii

INTRODUCTION   Evolution of the Sport of Bodybuilding   1

Early Physique Competitions   1
The Early 1900s   2
Pre–Golden Era   3
Golden Era   4
  ▸ Is it possible for bodybuilding competitors to compete
    in another strength sport (powerlifting, for example)?   4

The Late 20th Century   4

1   The Art and Science of Bodybuilding   7

New Divisions   7
Drug-Tested Bodybuilding   8
Misinformed Approaches to Contest Preparation   8
  ▸ Many competitors at my gym use methods you do not recommend yet
    have been successful in their competitions. Why should I follow the
    approaches discussed in this book rather than what the guys at my gym are doing?   10

2   Sorting Through the Sanctions   11

Drug Use in Bodybuilding   11
Untested Amateur Sanctions   12
  ▸ If I am drug-free, can I compete in untested competitions?   12

Untested Professional Sanctions   12
Drug-Tested Sanctions   12
  ▸ Are banned substances taken for diagnosed medical reasons allowed in drug-tested competitions?   13
  ▸ If I win a pro card in one sanction, can I compete in professional competitions in other sanctions?   13

3   Breaking Down the Divisions and Classes   15

Men's Divisions   15
Women's Divisions   22
  ▸ Can a competitor compete in more than one division at a show?   30

Final Word on Division Criteria   30
  ▸ I feel like I may be able to compete in more than one division. How do I choose the best division for me?   30

Classes   30
  ▸ Why are there multiple classes within the same show?
    For example, why are there three open men's bodybuilding classes?   31
  ▸ Can competitors make a living from prize money earned in professional competitions?   32
  ▸ Can a competitor compete in more than one class at a show?   33

4   The Reality of Readiness   35

New Competitors   35
- ▸ As a new competitor attending a competition for the first time, is it important for me to attend a competition in the sanction in which I plan to compete?   36

Experienced Competitors   37
- ▸ Would you ever recommend competing with less time between shows?   38

Readiness for Contest Prep   38
Patience and Time Pay Off   41

5   Show Selection and Timing: The Secrets of Preparation   43

Selecting the Right Show   43
- ▸ What is the best time for me to start contest prep?   44

Appropriate Rate of Loss   44
- ▸ Does my weight need to decrease to get stage-lean?   45

Benefits of Longer Prep Time   45
Determining Needed Prep Time   47
- ▸ Do I need to select a show before starting contest prep?   47
- ▸ Could I achieve stage-lean levels of body fat in less time than you recommend?   48

6   Fueling Your Physique for Contest Preparation   51

Energy Balance   51
Caloric Intake   52
- ▸ What do I do if I fall off my nutrition plan for a day?   54

Macronutrients   54
- ▸ Are high-protein diets safe?   56
- ▸ Should I be concerned about sugar intake during contest prep?   57

Individual Differences in Macronutrient Needs   58
- ▸ What is the best way to accurately measure my food?   59

Fiber   62
Vitamins and Minerals   63
- ▸ Can I have artificial sweeteners during contest prep?   64

Meal Frequency   64
Protein Timing   64
Carbohydrate Timing   65
Refeeds   66
Diet Breaks   67
Monitoring Progress   68
- ▸ How should a woman handle weight fluctuations due to her menstrual cycle?   68

Plateaus   69

7   Tweaking Your Physique for Contest Preparation   71

Increasing Energy Expenditure   71
  ► Should I do cardio fasted?   72
  ► If I am lifting weights and doing cardio in the same workout, which should I do first?   73

Resistance Training   74
  ► What is the mind-muscle connection I have heard about?   76
  ► How many days a week should I be in the gym?   77
  ► Do I need to train to failure? If so, should I do it in every workout?   78

Monitor the Need for Recovery   80
Sample Training Programs   80

8   The Art of Posing   91

Bodybuilding (Men and Women)   93
Classic Physique (Men)   94
Men's Physique   94
Women's Physique   94
Figure (Women)   95
Bikini (Women)   95
Posing Routines and T-Walks   170
Effective Practice Posing   170
  ► Should I practice the poses while wearing my posing suit?   171
  ► Should I pose in a sauna?   172

9   The Finishing Touches and Final Preparation   173

Posing Practice   173
Posing Music   173
Posing Suit   174
Shoes   174
Jewelry   174
Hair Removal   174
Tanning   175
  ► Do all competitions allow the same type of tan?   175
  ► Do I need to get a base tan in a tanning bed before my competition?   175

Makeup and Hair   176
Other Logistical Details   176
  ► When should I register for a show?   176

10 Peak Week Explained   179

Peak Week   179
Prerequisites for Effective Peaking   180
Terminology and Definitions   181
Peak Week Objectives   181
Peak Week Objective Nonstarters   182
Carbohydrates   183
Water   185
  ▸ Would you ever recommend that a competitor cut water during peak week?   187

Sodium-Potassium Balance   187
Peaking Network   189
Peak Week Strategies   189
Learning Your Load Look and Choosing a Peaking Strategy   196
Peak Week Training   196
Peak Week Cardio   197
Managing Your Physique on Show Day   198
  ▸ What if I mistime my sodium, sugar, and pump up backstage, and I am too early?   200

The Perfect Peak?   200

11 Contest Weekend: Strategizing for Success   201

Focus on What You Can Control   201
The Day Before the Show   202
Show Day   203
  ▸ How ready should I be when I arrive at the venue on show day?   204
  ▸ Can I go out to eat after prejudging?   205

After the Show   205

12 After the Event: Recovery and Recommendations   207

Postshow Analysis   207
Competing in Multiple Shows   207
Physiology of Being Stage-Lean   208
Transitioning to the Off-Season   209
  ▸ Does everyone need to regain body fat after a show?   211

Epilogue 213 • References 215 • Index 220 • About the Authors 222 • More Praise for *Bodybuilding* 224 •
Earn Continuing Education Credits/Units 226

FOREWORD

Because I am a competitor, I always like to see what kind of "secrets" will be revealed in books like this. (It's the nature of a bodybuilder, I guess!) I also look for how the explanations needed to give you your foundational knowledge are presented. Is the book understandable, or a collection of big words meant to impress you with how smart the authors are? I'm happy to say this book is easy to understand, and it does an incredible job of walking you through key concepts such as proper sodium and potassium levels, building metabolic capacity, protein requirements, and so on. I think it's a great reality check as well, as to costs associated with competing and the time it takes to build a championship physique. While this seems commonsense, it is not and needs to be discussed up front. I could go on and on about all the great concepts covered, but suffice to say this book gets two big thumbs up from me! Well done, Cliff and Peter!

—John Meadows

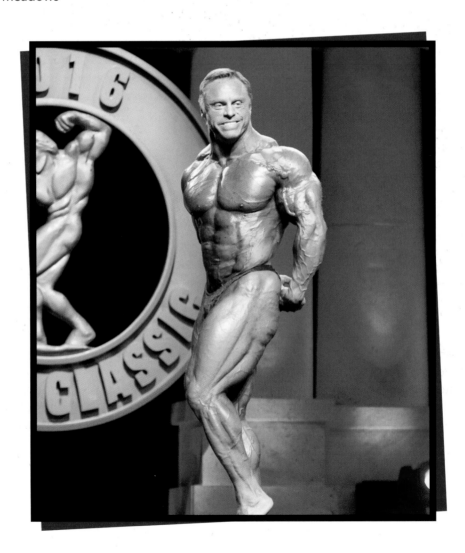

The popularity of bodybuilding is at an all-time high, and the sport is continuing to grow. This increase in the number of competitors has allowed both of us to work as full-time contest prep coaches. Throughout our careers, we have noticed similar questions from nearly every competitor. Some of these questions are about nutrition and training during contest preparation. Others are related to additional factors involved in competing, such as where to find shows, what type of tan to use, what happens on show day, and several other topics. These questions are not unique to beginners. Experienced competitors looking to improve their contest placing also ask these questions.

Currently, there is no single resource that sufficiently answers these questions in detail, so we answer many of the same questions repeatedly. Furthermore, many competitors do not work with an experienced coach who can provide this information. These individuals often rely on information they can find online or passed down in their gym. In many cases, this leads to sub-optimal approaches, a physique not ready to step onstage, and a poor placing.

This book provides a comprehensive overview of the bodybuilding contest process, from the start of preparation through show day and into the transition to the off-season.

The book is divided into three sections. The first focuses on bodybuilding background. When most people think of bodybuilding, they think of Arnold Schwarzenegger. The bodybuilding division that Arnold competed in is still a major part of the sport; however, several new competitive divisions are now offered at contests for both men and women. Discussion of these new divisions is a unique aspect of this book.

The second section of this book focuses on the process of obtaining a stage-ready physique. This section provides an evidence-based approach for contest preparation and combines scientific literature with our experience. In addition to discussing nutrition and training techniques, we give attention to important topics such as determining when a person is ready to begin preparing for a competition.

The final section covers many less-discussed aspects of contest preparation that add the finishing touches to a competitor's physique. This includes posing, peak week, tan, and several other topics that help a competitor bring a polished physique to the stage.

Another unique component to this book is that we discuss what to do after the show. Most resources on bodybuilding provide guidance on how to look the best onstage but rarely mention the postcontest period. As a result, many competitors are confused about this period and end up gaining significant amounts of body fat, which rapidly leads to physiological and psychological issues. Therefore, we provide detailed guidance on how to handle the period after a contest.

The content of this book is beneficial for any competitor, from beginner to advanced. Our goal is to provide a comprehensive approach to guide beginners through their first contests from start to finish. However, we also address less common topics to help an experienced competitor improve onstage. Ultimately, our goal is to make this book the most comprehensive guide to bodybuilding.

ACKNOWLEDGMENTS

A project of this magnitude would not have been possible without help from several people. Thank you to my coauthor, Cliff Wilson, for embarking on this journey with me. It has been a great experience collaborating with you on this project. I thank Human Kinetics for their support in all aspects of this project. Thank you also to all of the athletes and photographers who allowed us to use your images in our book.

Thank you to everyone who, early in my training career, took time to answer questions from a 125-pound, inquisitive teenager looking to learn more about bodybuilding. Thanks to Dr. Layne Norton for being a mentor to me early in my bodybuilding career and getting me interested in the science of bodybuilding. I also thank my advisors in graduate school, Dr. Margaret Maher and Dr. Kenneth Wilund, for all their knowledge and support during my formal education.

To all my clients over the years, thank you for putting your trust in me as your coach. Without you, none of this would have been possible. This book is the product of my experiences working with all of you.

I thank my wife, Amy, for supporting my endeavors in academics, bodybuilding, and coaching and the long hours associated with writing this book. Thanks to all my family and friends, both inside and outside the bodybuilding world. I greatly appreciate the support you have given me and could not have done this without you.

—Peter J. Fitschen, PhD, CSCS

The results of this book are the product of the hours that went into writing it and the years that allowed me to obtain all the information and experience I needed to write it. For that reason, I need to thank many people for helping my growth and development. First, I need to thank my coauthor, Peter Fitschen. You have been not only a great colleague but also a great friend. It has been a pleasure creating this with you.

I want to thank Katie Wilson for all she has done for me over the years to help me become who I am today, trusting in my vision and always having faith in me. You always supported me and had faith in what I was trying to do. None of this would have been possible without you.

To my dad for being a constant source of wisdom and council, to my mom for always believing in my abilities, and to my grandma for always giving selflessly to make sure I was not in need. I am eternally grateful. Thank you to my little brother, Chad, for being not only a great source of motivation but also a great friend as you have grown.

Thank you to Haley Clevenger for being my support system while I put in long hours finishing this book, caring for me even when I forget to care for myself and putting me back on track to being the man I know I am capable of being.

I also need to thank all the clients who have ever put their trust in me as a coach, particularly those who trusted me early in my career when I was still a very unproven commodity. It is because of you that I can do what I love every day.

—Cliff Wilson

PHOTO CREDITS

Evolution of the Sport of Bodybuilding

Bodybuilding as we know it today developed from the long history of weightlifting. The first gymnasiums were established in ancient Greece. These gyms were significantly different than modern gyms. Athletes primarily trained for the events in which they competed as opposed to training for muscle size. There is also record that in India, as far back as the 11th century, dumbbell-like weights made of stone were lifted by those looking to enhance health and strength. This goes to show how instinctual it is for human beings to gravitate toward developing strength and athletic ability.

In the 19th century, it was believed that individuals would become "muscle bound" to the point where their muscles would literally lock up if they got too big. Despite this pervasive mainstream belief, strongman events gained popularity. These events typically involved two men challenging each other at various feats of strength. Events ranged from things like lifting weights and stones to pulling carts and even lifting animals. There were no real sanctions or awards for these events. Strongmen would travel from town to town challenging other strongmen often with nothing more than pride as the prize. However, these types of competitions remained popular until around the 1930s.

The winner of these events was the man who lifted more weight. Physiques were not judged, and the average strongman did not have a physique like bodybuilders stepping onstage today. Competitors did not focus on diet, and as a result, strongmen had relatively high body fat percentages.

EARLY PHYSIQUE COMPETITIONS

Eugene Sandow was the first professional strongman who looked different than the rest. Unlike other strongmen of the time, he focused on his diet and paid attention to what he ate. As a result, he was leaner, had more muscle definition, and looked more like what we would consider a bodybuilder today. Along with competing in strongman events, he also began doing muscle exhibitions that resemble today's posing routines. Over his career, he traveled around the world and created an industry around building a physique. He sold barbells and dumbbells and is credited with developing the first exercise machine. He also created *Magazine of Physical Culture* that focused on building a muscular physique.

Later in his career, he began hosting competitions where men would compete based on physical appearance in addition to feats of strength. In 1901, he hosted the Great Competition at Royal Albert Hall in London. Sandow advertised the competition for three years in his magazine, and competitors had to have placed in a regional event to compete. Competitors wore a black jockey belt, black tights, and leopard skins, a far cry from the posing trunks worn onstage today.

The Great Competition winner received the equivalent of $5,000 at the time and a gold trophy cast with an image of Sandow himself. The second- and third-place winners received a silver and bronze trophy, respectively. Interestingly, the Sandow trophy given to the Mr. Olympia winner today is a bronze replica of the trophy given to the third-place Great Competition winner. It is said that the gold trophy was destroyed during the World Wars; however, the bronze statue resurfaced as a prize for the 1950 Mr. Universe competition in London and was won by Steve Reeves, an American. The trophy would not be used again until a replica was given to the 1977 International Federation of Bodybuilding and Fitness (IFBB) Mr. Olympia competition winner. Each Mr. Olympia winner since has received a replica of the bronze Sandow Trophy given to the third-place winner at the Great Competition in 1901.

While Eugene Sandow was starting the physical culture movement in the United Kingdom, Bernarr MacFadden was doing the same in the United States. In 1904 he promoted the "most perfectly developed man in the world" competition at Madison Square Garden in New York with a prize of $1,000. Like the competitions Sandow was promoting, McFadden's competitions required athletes to lift heavy objects in addition to having their physiques judged onstage.

THE EARLY 1900s

During the early 1900s, knowledge about building muscle and bodybuilding was still in its infancy, but many were realizing that weightlifting could play a large role in sculpting a muscular and lean physique. The number of competitions increased, and these competitions required both athletic events as well as visual or physique components. Charles Atlas was the most famous bodybuilder in the world during this time and was widely featured in the *Magazine of Physical Culture*.

Unlike today, where bodybuilders lift weights to prepare for competition, competitors came from a variety of backgrounds such as wrestling, gymnastics, or weightlifting. However, it was becoming increasingly clear that weightlifters were placing higher in these competitions. As a result, by the 1920s, barbells, dumbbells, and other exercise devices were sold around the world. By the 1930s, the number of gyms began to increase as well.

In the early years of competitions, competitors were asked to perform a wide array of "lifts" (often called *exercises*), but very few records were kept of poundage moved in competition. However, in 1911 the British Amateur Weightlifting Association was founded to begin collecting records for 42 different lifts. These lifts included the deadlift, overhead press, supine press (an early version of a bench press where the athlete lay on the ground), deep-knee bend (an extremely deep squat often performed for reps), upright row, several single-arm dumbbell lifts, and many others. In the United States, similar organizations formed over the next two decades to begin registering records.

In 1920, the number of lifts primarily performed in strength competitions were reduced when Olympic weightlifting was limited to three main lifts: snatch, overhead press, and clean and jerk. All the other lifts became known as the odd lifts. The early versions of the big three (squat, bench, and deadlift) performed in powerlifting meets today were considered odd lifts. Many bodybuilders still used many of the odd lifts in training and included exhibitions of them at competition, although these lifts were not included in Olympic weightlifting.

PRE–GOLDEN ERA

The period between 1940 and the mid to late 1960s is often called the pre–golden era or silver era of bodybuilding because it precedes the golden era (the late 1960s through early 1980s). The start of this period is often considered the 1940 American Athletic Union (AAU) Mr. America competition, referred to as the first real modern bodybuilding event. Competitors in the Mr. America competed in both weightlifting and posing. For an athlete to win, he needed to excel in both endeavors. The weightlifting component heavily focused on the Olympic lifts at this time.

Muscle beach also became popular in the 1940s. It was an outdoor gym where athletes lifted weights, did gymnastics, and performed strength events such as bending steel rods and tearing phone books as people watched. There was also an increase in the number of beach contests consisting of a combination of bodybuilding, strength competitions, and gymnastics along the coasts of Southern California.

Most competitors of this era trained only three days a week (Mondays, Wednesdays, and Fridays) because these were often the only days the gym was open. Workouts were full body each day, with each muscle group trained three times weekly. Some gyms during this period were open to women on Tuesdays, Thursdays, and Saturdays. However, this was a period of gender segregation for physical fitness and exercise. In fact, many major universities at this time had separate gymnasiums for men and women. (This includes the University of Illinois; during Peter's graduate studies there, his research lab was in the former women's physical fitness building.)

Steve Reeves was the most famous bodybuilder during this period and is considered the first truly well-known bodybuilder. Reeves was a successful competitor, winning the 1947 Mr. America, 1948 Mr. World, and 1950 Mr. Universe; however, his fame came from the movies he starred in, such as *Hercules*. His aesthetic physique and good looks made him popular with a more mainstream crowd.

This was also when bodybuilders primarily competed drug-free. The first confirmed use of steroids in strength sports was at the 1954 World Weightlifting Competition in Vienna, Austria, by the Soviet weightlifting team. However, Dianabol, a commonly used anabolic steroid, did not become available until 1958 and did not begin to appear in bodybuilding circles until the 1960s. Many mark this appearance of drug use within the sport as the end of the pre–golden era of bodybuilding.

As a side note, people today are quick to accuse anyone with a more developed physique of using performance-enhancing drugs; however, the high-level physiques developed without drugs before the 1950s and 1960s clearly show what can be accomplished naturally. There were some impressive physiques during this period even though diet and training methods are not as advanced as today. Both authors encourage readers to focus on their own progress and goals rather than spending time worrying about what others are or are not taking to enhance their physiques.

By the 1950s, bodybuilding popularity was increasing, as were the number of gyms, but interest in Olympic weightlifting was declining. As a result, the AAU (which previously focused primarily on Olympic lifts in competition) started recording odd lift records in 1958. The first powerlifting meet was held in 1964, and the first national championship was held the following year. The three lifts selected for these meets were a deep-knee bend variation in which a competitor only squatted to parallel, a supine press variation performed on a bench rather than the ground, and the classic deadlift that has remained relatively unchanged.

The number of sanctions and competitions also increased during this time. The AAU, IFBB, and the National Amateur Bodybuilding Association (NABBA) were just a few of the many sanctions that battled for competitors. Each sanction had a most prestigious title, such as the Mr. America or Mr. Universe; however, no competition definitively determined the best bodybuilder in the world. That all changed when Joe Weider promoted the IFBB Mr. Olympia in 1965, ushering in the golden era of bodybuilding.

GOLDEN ERA

The beginning of the golden era of bodybuilding is typically marked as either the introduction of drug use into the sport or the first Mr. Olympia competition, both of which occurred around the mid-1960s. During this period, the popularity of bodybuilding skyrocketed, and the profitability of gyms increased, leading to more gyms dedicated to bodybuilders. In 1965, Joe Gold opened the first Gold's Gym in Venice Beach, California. Since then, Gold's Gym has been franchised to over 700 locations, and many other successful gym franchises have also emerged.

This was also the time when the iconic documentary *Pumping Iron* was filmed. This introduced a wide audience to Arnold Schwarzenegger and other top bodybuilders of the time, such as Lou Ferrigno and Franco Columbo. As a result, the sport's popularity grew massively.

During this period, bodybuilding competitions also began to change. Unlike bodybuilders of previous eras, golden-era bodybuilders began to be judged on appearance alone and no longer had to also perform athletic events in competition. Powerlifting, Olympic weightlifting, and strongman became separate competitions and allowed competitors to specialize in their goals.

FAQ: Is it possible for bodybuilding competitors to compete in another strength sport (powerlifting, for example)?

Many bodybuilders compete in other strength sports in the off-season. Competing in a strength sport like powerlifting allows the athlete to focus on heavy compound movements that can be a great way for a bodybuilder to add muscle mass. However, we would encourage bodybuilders who also compete in powerlifting (or another strength sport like Olympic lifting or strongman) to add assistance exercises to their training to ensure each muscle group is being targeted with enough volume to build a symmetrical physique.

The ideal physique of the golden era was a large *V* taper with wide shoulders, big arms, and big lats that tapered down to a tiny waist. Bodybuilders like Arnold Schwarzenegger (Mr. America, five-time Mr. Universe, and seven-time Mr. Olympia) and Frank Zane (Mr. America, three-time Mr. Universe, and three-time Mr. Olympia) were the epitome of this aesthetic look. To achieve this look, training transitioned from three weekly full-body workouts to five to six days a week training a single body part daily with high training volumes.

During this period, the IFBB's Mr. Olympia competition began to dominate the competition scene. Bodybuilders wanted to become the best in the world and that meant winning the IFBB Mr. Olympia. In 1981, the National Physique Committee (NPC) formed as an amateur affiliate to the IFBB. As a result, most of the other competing sanctions gradually died off and the NPC/IFBB remains the primary untested bodybuilding sanction to this date.

THE LATE 20TH CENTURY

As bodybuilding entered the 1980s, the sport began to change. Drug use increased, and the physiques onstage became larger as the focus of the *V* taper began to fade. Many mark the end of the golden era of bodybuilding as 1984 when Lee Haney won his first Mr. Olympia title. He would go on to win eight consecutive Mr. Olympia titles from 1984 to 1991.

What made Haney different is that he was significantly larger than previous Mr. Olympia winners at 5'11" (180 cm) and 240 to 245 pounds (109-111 kg). In comparison, the Mr. Olympia winners of the golden age were smaller: Arnold Schwarzenegger (6'2" [188 cm], 225 to 230 pounds [102-104 kg]), Frank Zane (5'9" [175 cm], 185 pounds [84 kg]), and Franco Columbo (5'5" [165 cm], 185 pounds [84 kg]). Haney's successors to the Mr. Olympia throne, Dorian Yates (1992-1997) and Ronnie Coleman (1998-2005), only continued to increase in size. Yates was 265 pounds (120 kg) onstage at 5'10" (178 cm), and Coleman at his largest was nearly 300 pounds (136 kg) onstage at 5'11" (180 cm). By the end of the century, bodybuilding in the IFBB had primarily become a mass game.

The sport of bodybuilding continued to expand during this time. A number of women entered the sport, and the first Ms. Olympia was held in 1980. In 1989, Arnold created the Arnold Classic, which has become the second most prestigious title in the IFBB and the largest fitness expo in the United States.

In 1990, the U.S. government made anabolic steroids a class III substance. Around this time, the interest in drug-tested bodybuilding increased. By the end of the century, several new sanctions, such as the International Natural Bodybuilding Association (INBA), National Gym Association (NGA), and World Natural Bodybuilding Federation (WNBF) began to provide alternative options to competitors who chose to compete without using drugs. Heading into the 21st century, the popularity of bodybuilding continued to increase as the opportunities to compete increased.

Take-Home Points

► Bodybuilding competitions initially developed from muscle exhibitions that accompanied strongman competitions. However, these strongman competitions were different from strongman competitions today and typically involved one strongman challenging another in various feats of strength.

► Early bodybuilding competitions involved an athletic performance component along with a physique component. Depending on the competition, the athletic component had Olympic weightlifting, gymnastics, or odd lifts, including early versions of the big three powerlifting lifts. Competitors needed to excel at both components to win the competitions.

► By the golden age of bodybuilding, physique competitions no longer included an athletic component, and athletes were solely judged on visual appearance. Powerlifting, Olympic weightlifting, and strongman became separate competitions.

► The desired look of a bodybuilder before the early 1980s was a large *V* taper, small waist, and very aesthetic look. However, by the turn of the century, professional bodybuilding in the IFBB had become a mass game.

► The popularity of bodybuilding grew throughout the 20th century. By the end of the century, there were competitions for women and for those who chose to compete drug-free. As a result, more people than ever before were competing in bodybuilding.

The Art and Science of Bodybuilding

In the introduction, our discussion of bodybuilding history left off around the turn of the century, when Mr. Olympia competitors were becoming larger and heavier. While "mass monsters" like Ronnie Coleman and Jay Cutler dominated the early part of the 21st century, this led to the development of new divisions, and a large influx in competitors as the sport expressed an increased desire for a more streamlined and aesthetic look. This change can be seen in the physiques of more recent Mr. Olympia winners and top contenders; fewer were around the 300-pound (136 kg) mark onstage. For example, the physiques of 2008 Mr. Olympia Dexter Jackson (5' 6" [168 cm], 215 pounds [98 kg]), the seven-time Mr. Olympia Phil Heath (5' 9" [175 cm], 240 pounds [109 kg]), and 2018 Mr. Olympia Shawn Rhoden (5' 10" [175cm], 240 pounds [109 kg]) are a stark contrast to the prior era when the mass monsters were king.

NEW DIVISIONS

The increasing desire for more aesthetic physiques also resulted in several new divisions. In 2008, the IFBB began to include a 202-pound (92 kg) pro class that was increased to be the 212-pound (96 kg) pro class in 2012.

In 2011, the NPC/IFBB introduced the men's physique division, where competitors are expected to have muscle mass. However, physiques that are too muscular are marked down. Similarly, competitors are expected to be extremely lean, but competitors with overly striated and vascular muscle are marked down. Competitors in this division wear board shorts and are primarily judged from the waist up.

As the demand for a more streamlined look in bodybuilding continued to increase, the classic physique division was added in 2016. This division was meant to serve as a middle ground between the physiques in the men's physique and the men's bodybuilding divisions. Successful competitors in the classic physique division have an aesthetic physique, large *V* taper, and a similar look to bodybuilders of the golden age, but they are typically leaner than competitors of the golden age. The classic physique division also has weight limits based on a competitor's height to encourage a more aesthetic physique.

Male competitors are not the only ones with new divisions in the 21st century. The women's side of the sport has also seen rapid expansion. The new women's divisions are less extreme than the women's bodybuilding division to encourage more females to compete. The first division added was figure. The first national event was in 2001, and the first professional event was in 2003. Women in this division are less muscular and not as striated as female bodybuilders. They also wear high heels and jewelry and are, in part, judged on femininity. This attracted female competitors who enjoyed weight training but did not want to push the limits of their muscularity too far.

In 2010, the NPC/IFBB added the bikini division. Competitors in this division were less muscular and conditioned than figure competitors were. However, like the figure division, competitors wear heels and jewelry, and femininity is a judged component. In contrast, posing is less rigid than the figure division, and competitors can show a bit more personality onstage. The bikini division has quickly become the most popular women's division offered.

In 2011, the women's physique division was added. This division fits between the figure and bodybuilding divisions in terms of muscularity and conditioning. Competitors do not wear heels in the physique division, but the posing is more stereotypically feminine than in the bodybuilding division.

With the addition of two new male and three new female divisions, competitors now have more divisions to best suit their physiques. The judging criteria and posing for each division will be discussed in chapters 3 and 8, respectively.

DRUG-TESTED BODYBUILDING

Over the past two decades, the number of drug-tested bodybuilding competitions has increased exponentially. This has increased the number of overall competitors in the sport by providing a level playing field for those who choose to compete without the use of drugs. Competitors in drug-tested competitions are typically polygraph- and urine-tested. In addition, some sanctions perform random off-season testing for professional drug-tested athletes.

With the increase in competitors participating in drug-tested shows, many new sanctions have started to offer competitions. In 2018, over 300 drug-tested competitions were scheduled in the United States. However, these are scattered across more than a dozen sanctions. In comparison, the NPC (the primary non-tested amateur bodybuilding sanction in the United States) had over 200 competitions in 2018 alone.

Each drug-tested bodybuilding sanction has its own professional competition serving as the most prestigious title. Examples include the WNBF Worlds, IPE Worlds, OCB Yorton Cup, NGA Universe, PNBA Natural Olympia, and several others. Chapter 2 includes a detailed list of bodybuilding sanctions.

The current state of drug-tested bodybuilding in the United States is like bodybuilding during the pre–golden era, before the first IFBB Mr. Olympia in 1965. The sport's growth has resulted in several new sanctions, competitions, and many new competitors, but there is no unity within the sport. However, there is a strong call from competitors for more unity and a hope that drug-tested bodybuilding can one day develop a more uniform structure like the NPC/IFBB.

MISINFORMED APPROACHES TO CONTEST PREPARATION

Historically, information about preparing for a bodybuilding contest was passed down from competitor to competitor at the gym. Little scientific research had been performed on bodybuilders preparing for competition, and before the Internet, there was no realistic way for most competitors to access this information even if it had existed. Much published research tests the approaches that bodybuilders have been using for decades. Some approaches have withstood the test of time, others have been disproven, and many have simply not been tested in a research setting but appear to be effective in practice.

Previously, most bodybuilders would prepare (simply called *prep*) for a standard of 8 to 12 weeks regardless of how much fat they needed to lose. This was the way people had "always done things," so most people followed this plan. Sixteen-week preps were considered long contest preps, and prep times of more than 20 weeks were almost unheard of (4). However, research (2) and anecdotal evidence suggest there may be many advantages to a longer prep time. In fact, this is such a common misconception among competitors that we dedicated an entire chapter (chapter 5) to discussing how long to plan for an effective contest prep.

Once contest prep started, competitors would often follow set meal plans, eating the same thing each day. Even in the early 2000s, when we began competing, this approach was extremely common.

A contest prep meal plan could look like the following:

- ▶ Meal 1: egg whites, oatmeal
- ▶ Meal 2: chicken breast, green vegetables
- ▶ Meal 3 (preworkout): chicken breast, sweet potato
- ▶ Meal 4 (immediately postworkout): protein shake
- ▶ Meal 5: tilapia, brown rice, green vegetables
- ▶ Meal 6: lean beef, green vegetables

For either a meal or an entire day each week, a competitor would have a "cheat meal" or "cheat day" when he or she could consume anything desired.

Although there are many problems with this nutritional approach, one of the most glaring issues is that it was completely normal for a bodybuilder to eliminate dairy and fruit from the diet during contest prep. As a result, nutritional deficiencies were common, with the most typical being calcium and vitamin D (4). Another issue with such a diet plan is that on cheat days competitors often undid all the progress that was made during the week by consuming too many calories. If you are looking at the sample meal plan and thinking there is no way you could follow it, do not assume that competing is not for you—an approach this extreme is not only unnecessary, it is also not as effective as a more moderate approach. Chapter 6 will discuss how to modify your nutrition for an effective contest prep.

While traditional bodybuilding dietary approaches have been wrought with issues, training was no different. It was completely normal for competitors to switch to exclusively high repetitions during contest prep due to the belief that this "tones" the muscle. However, this approach commonly results in strength and muscle loss during contest prep (1). Long durations of steady-state fasted cardio first thing in the morning were also commonplace, as were cardio durations of more than 10 hours weekly (7). However, neither of these may be necessary or optimal to develop a stage-ready physique based on more research (3), observation, and experience. We will cover resistance training and cardio for contest prep in detail in chapter 7.

The final week before a competition is commonly called **peak week**. In this final week, competitors often take extreme approaches to drastically alter their physiques, including cutting water and sodium (4). However, these approaches may make a competitor's physique look worse come show day (2). Chapter 10 describes more effective approaches to peak week.

After a competition, rapid weight gain was common (5). However, research suggests that gaining weight too rapidly may add to excessive fat gain and slow the return of hormones to normal levels (6). Therefore, chapter 12 covers how to transition out of a competition, what to do in the off-season, and why an off-season is important.

Through the approaches outlined in this book, our goal is to provide comprehensive guidelines for contest prep based on research and our experience as competitors and coaches.

FAQ: Many competitors at my gym use methods you do not recommend yet have been successful in their competitions. Why should I follow the approaches discussed in this book rather than what the guys at my gym are doing?

A person can use many approaches during contest prep, and some will be more successful than others. There is no way to tell whether a different approach may have worked better for the competitors at your gym. We encourage all competitors to test a variety of approaches to find what works best for them; however, we would encourage using the evidence-based approaches described in this book as a starting point to developing a stage-ready physique. The recommendations provided are a combination of our experience as coaches and competitors as well as scientific research.

Take-Home Points

► In recent years, bodybuilding has had a large increase in competitors due to several new divisions for both men (men's physique and classic physique) and women (figure, bikini, and women's physique).

► Drug-tested bodybuilding has grown in recent years, giving competitors who choose to compete drug-free an option for a level playing field during competition.

► Studies show many common contest prep practices are unnecessary or suboptimal.

Sorting Through the Sanctions

It does not matter if you are new to bodybuilding or a seasoned competitor; choosing a bodybuilding sanction can be confusing. The growth of bodybuilding has led to many new sanctions, and they seem to change every few years. To complicate things further, some sanctions drug test while others do not. It can be especially difficult for a new competitor to know the difference between the sanctions. Even within drug-tested sanctions, testing policies may also differ, and that can make things even more confusing.

In addition, new competitors may not understand the difference between professional and amateur competitions and who is eligible to compete at each. The process of obtaining professional status differs between sanctions. Some sanctions may accept a competitor's professional status from another sanction while others do not.

This chapter helps you sort through the sanctions so you can select the competition best for you.

DRUG USE IN BODYBUILDING

While it is a taboo subject, **performance-enhancing drugs** (PEDs) have been a part of bodybuilding for over 60 years. It is important to address drug use before discussing the differences in drug testing between sanctions since it plays into choosing the bodybuilding federation that best suits you.

What a competitor puts in his or her body is ultimately his or her own decision. We do not discourage or endorse drug use in this book but want to help both those who use drugs and those who do not learn what their options are in terms of choosing a sanction. Individuals considering using PEDs should discuss this decision with a physician or qualified medical professional. We encourage those using PEDs to have routine bloodwork performed by a qualified health professional.

We will not discuss protocols for using PEDs in this book. However, all other contest prep approaches will be applicable, regardless of the sanction chosen.

UNTESTED AMATEUR SANCTIONS

The NPC is the primary untested amateur bodybuilding sanction in the United States, and it has over 200 scheduled competitions. Information about the NPC and its competitions can be found at www.npcnewsonline.com.

Competitors within the NPC do not need to qualify for regional amateur competitions, but amateur competitors do not win prize money. However, competitors can become NPC nationally qualified based on placing at a regional show. At designated national qualifying competitions, if a male competitor places in the top two or a female competitor places in the top three of the open division, he or she becomes nationally qualified. There may be other situations when a competitor qualifies as well. Consult with the NPC website or NPC show promoters with specific questions regarding national qualification.

When a competitor becomes nationally qualified, he or she is eligible to compete at national-level NPC competitions for one year. Examples of these competitions include NPC Nationals, NPC Junior Nationals, NPC Universe, NPC USA, and others. Competitors at national competitions can be awarded professional status in the IFBB based on placing. Many competitors want to turn pro and compete in the IFBB. Much like in other athletic endeavors, turning pro is extremely difficult because the competition is stiff. The number of IFBB pro cards awarded differs between competitions. Consult with the show information for each specific national-level show for more information regarding obtaining professional status in the IFBB.

FAQ: If I am drug-free, can I compete in untested competitions?

Yes, competitors who are drug-free can compete in untested competitions. Competitors in untested competitions are often taking substances that a drug-free athlete is not. However, it is well within the competition rules, and a drug-free athlete should not blame placing in an untested competition on drug use by other competitors.

UNTESTED PROFESSIONAL SANCTIONS

The IFBB is the primary untested professional bodybuilding sanction worldwide, and it promotes competitions such as the Mr. Olympia, Arnold Classic, and many others. IFBB Mr. Olympia winners are usually considered the best in the world in their divisions.

As previously discussed, competitors in the United States can qualify through the NPC. However, international competitors can also qualify through amateur sanctions in their countries and should consult with those sanctions for details about how to obtain professional status. More information about the IFBB can be found at www.ifbb.com.

DRUG-TESTED SANCTIONS

Through most of bodybuilding history, competitions have not been drug tested. However, as drug use has become more prevalent in the past two or three decades, the demand for drug-tested shows has increased dramatically. As a result, many bodybuilding sanctions test athletes before competition, usually through polygraph and urine testing. Some sanctions have also moved toward off-season testing of professional drug-free competitors. While there is only one primary untested bodybuilding sanction (NPC/IFBB), there are currently many drug-tested federations to choose from.

Although the banned substance lists differ between sanctions, the substances that are typically banned are anabolic steroids, growth hormones, thyroid hormone, insulin, ephedra, clenbuterol, prescription diuretics (herbal diuretics are typically legal for use), and any other substance that raises testosterone levels above the physiological range. To avoid issues, we encourage all competitors considering a drug-tested competition to consult the banned substance list before signing up. The primary differences in the banned substance lists of different sanctions are regarding certain over-the-counter supplements as well as the use of physician-monitored hormone replacement therapy. Just because a supplement is sold legally over the counter, that does not mean it is automatically allowed in all drug-tested federations. For this reason, it's important to check with your sanction's guidelines before you use any new supplement.

FAQ: Are banned substances taken for diagnosed medical reasons allowed in drug-tested competitions?

Most drug-tested sanctions do not allow testosterone replacement therapy. Thyroid hormone and diuretics prescribed for a medical condition may be allowed. When in doubt, contact your sanction before registering for the competition to avoid any issues.

Like the NPC, a competitor does not have to qualify for an amateur competition. Also, just as in the NPC, prize money is not awarded in these contests. Unlike the NPC, competitors do not need to compete at national events to obtain pro status. Competitors can obtain professional status in a drug-tested sanction by winning the open overall in their divisions at a competition designated as a pro qualifier. Once a competitor obtains professional status in a drug-tested sanction, he or she can compete in drug-tested professional competitions for prize money. At this point, most drug-tested sanctions accept a competitor's professional status won in another sanction; however, we recommend asking the sanction in which you plan to compete if there are any questions.

FAQ: If I win a pro card in one sanction, can I compete in professional competitions in other sanctions?

Most drug-tested sanctions honor the professional status obtained in other drug-tested sanctions. However, the IFBB will not honor pro status obtained in a drug-tested sanction. We encourage those who have questions regarding professional eligibility to contact the sanction where they plan to compete for clarification.

Table 2.1 provides information about many amateur and professional drug-tested sanctions. Some smaller sanctions may be omitted. Also, the table does not include international sanctions. The landscape of drug-tested bodybuilding has undergone many changes over the years; however, all affiliations and links listed below are up-to-date at the time this book was written.

Table 2.1 Drug-Tested Bodybuilding Sanctions in the United States

SANCTION	WEBSITE	PROFESSIONAL AFFILIATE	MOST PRESTIGIOUS PROFESSIONAL TITLE	DRUG-TESTING POLICY
American Natural Bodybuilding Federation (ANBF)	www.anbfnatural.com	ANBF	ANBF World Championships	7 years drug-free; WADA testing
Drug Free Athletes Coalition (DFAC)	www.drugfreeathletes coalition.com	DFAC	DFAC World Finals	7 years drug-free; WADA testing
International Natural Bodybuilding Association (INBA)	http://naturalbodybuild ing.com	PNBA	PNBA Natural Olympia	5 years drug-free; IOC-regulated standards
International Natural Bodybuilding Federation (INBF)	www.worldnaturalbb.com	WNBF	WNBF World Championships	7 years drug-free; WADA testing
National Gym Association (NGA)	www.nationalgym.com	NGA	NGA Universe	7 years drug-free; IOC-banned substance list
North American Natural Bodybuilding Federation (NANBF)	http://nanbf.org	IPE	IPE World Championships	7 years drug-free
Organization of Competitive Bodybuilders (OCB)	http://ocboline.com	OCB	OCB Yorton Cup	7 years drug-free; WADA testing
World Physique Alliance (WPA)	www.worldphysiquealli ance.com	IPE	IPE World Championships	7 years drug-free

Take-Home Points

► The primary amateur and professional untested sanctions in the United States are the NPC and IFBB, respectively. The most prestigious title in the IFBB is Mr. Olympia.

► Currently, there are many drug-tested bodybuilding sanctions. Most sanctions have similar drug-testing policies; however, it is always best to research the sanction you plan to compete in before entering a competition.

► Amateur competitors in untested or drug-tested competitions typically do not have to qualify; however, competitors do not receive prize money. To win prize money in a competition, competitors must obtain professional status and place in a professional competition.

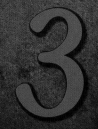

Breaking Down the Divisions and Classes

In the late 1990s, deciding which division to compete in at a bodybuilding competition was easy. If you were a man, you competed in men's bodybuilding, and if you were a woman, you competed in women's bodybuilding. In the early 2000s, several new divisions were added. This positive change provides options for competitors based on preferences and strengths, but it can make choosing a division more confusing.

We will clear up some of the confusion by explaining how the three criteria—muscularity, conditioning, and symmetry (see the Criteria Defined section at the end of the chapter for definitions)—are judged in each division. The ideal look for each division differs.

Division Finder

NAME	PAGE NUMBER
Men's bodybuilding	16
Classic physique	18
Men's physique	20
Women's bodybuilding	22
Women's physique	24
Figure	26
Bikini	28

MEN'S DIVISIONS

Men can enter the bodybuilding, classic physique, and physique divisions. Each differs from the other two based on the criteria for muscularity, conditioning and muscular definition, and symmetry.

Men's Bodybuilding

Muscularity   The criteria for muscularity in men's bodybuilding are simple: the more muscle, the better. Muscle size is a primary factor for winning a bodybuilding show.

Conditioning and Muscular Definition   Conditioning in men's bodybuilding is the most extreme of all divisions: you want to get as lean as possible. However, do not pursue fat loss to the point that you sacrifice muscularity. Proper dietary, cardio, and training methods ensure maximum fat loss and maximum muscle retention.

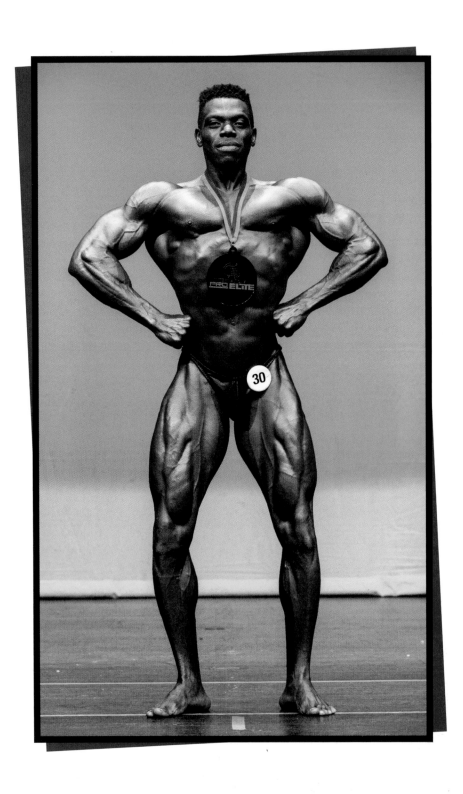

Symmetry   The standard for muscular symmetry in men's bodybuilding is to have an even balance of development among all muscle groups. For structural symmetry, it is ideal to have wide-set shoulders and a small waist.

Additional Considerations   The competitors in men's bodybuilding wear posing trunks. In today's competitive landscape, competitors wear trunks that show some glute muscle. The days when you could leave something to the imagination are gone, unfortunately.

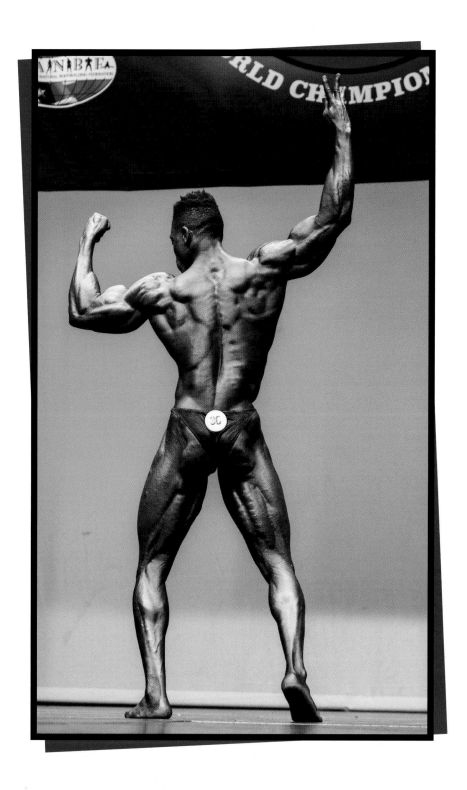

Classic Physique

Muscularity   Classic physique would best be described as requiring slightly less muscularity than in bodybuilding. But both authors find that it is rare to find any drug-free male who can achieve a look that would be considered too muscular for this division, so most men should train for maximum muscularity. For competitors who use PEDs, it is indeed possible to become too large if you are not careful, so do not push things too far.

Conditioning and Muscular Definition   In regard to conditioning, the classic physique division calls for a look that is slightly less lean than in bodybuilding. However, in practice, we often see the leanest competitors place higher. Do not get so lean that you sacrifice fullness. Because the glutes do not show in classic physique posing trunks, striated glutes are not necessary. This means if your

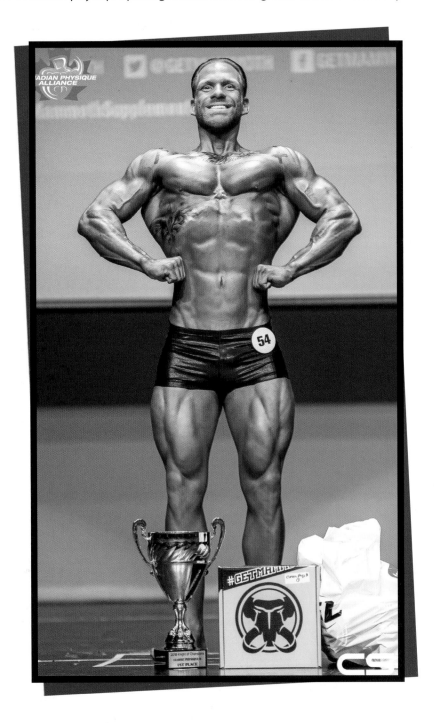

glutes are the last area to lean out, you may want to stop just short of seeing visible glute striations in order to preserve fullness in the other muscle groups.

Symmetry   The criteria for muscular symmetry in classic physique are to have an even balance of development among all muscle groups. For structural symmetry, it is ideal to have wide-set shoulders and a small waist.

Additional Considerations   Competitors in classic physique must wear posing trunks similar to bike shorts. As mentioned, they should cover your glutes and the top of your upper quads. Although classic physique has a different look in terms of muscle size for nondrug-tested shows, in drug-tested shows, classic physique looks nearly identical to bodybuilding except that competitors wear different posing trunks.

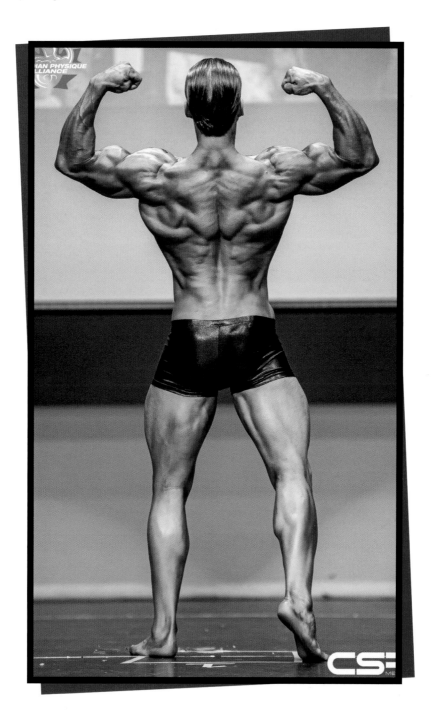

Men's Physique

Muscularity   Unlike in the bodybuilding division, it is possible to be too muscular in men's physique. How muscular is too muscular? This is the challenge. Different judges and different shows commonly have varied ideals for how muscular a physique athlete should be. Most competitors will have the best results by continuing to strive for more muscle mass. While it is technically possible to be too muscular, most drug-free competitors do not reach this level. Our best advice is to continue to train for as much muscle as possible; if the judges tell you that you are too muscular, then you can scale back your training a bit. If you are a drug-using competitor, slowly build up, and do not push things too far too quickly.

Conditioning and Muscular Definition   Many sanctions claim that men's physique competitors should not be too shredded, but this does not always reflect real-life competition. Our experience as coaches has shown us that leaner is usually better, and many more successful physique competitors are almost every bit as lean as bodybuilders. Our recommendation is to get as lean as possible but stop just short of seeing striations in your glute muscle.

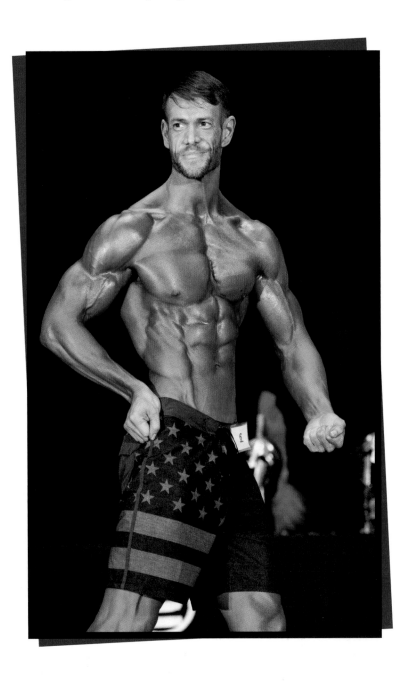

Symmetry   In men's physique, it is favorable to be most developed in the heavily judged muscle groups: abdominals, pectorals, delts, back, biceps, triceps, and calves. It is not necessary to fully develop the quads, hamstrings, or glutes. Although muscularity of these areas is a good thing, there is no need to aim for maximum development since they are not judged. The ideal men's physique competitor will also have a small waist and wide-set shoulders.

Additional Considerations   Men's physique competitors wear board shorts similar to a swimsuit. It covers your quads, hamstrings, and glutes, so those areas are not judged.

Competitors who are not very muscular may think they must belong in men's physique rather than in bodybuilding. However, this is not always the case. In men's physique, you have fewer ways to beat your opponent because there are only four poses. In bodybuilding, there are 13 poses, meaning there are more ways to pose to your advantage. Also, leg conditioning and muscularity are not considered in physique, so there are even fewer ways to gain an advantage if your genetics give you a body type with features judged unfavorably in this division. If you are smaller but have well-developed legs, it may be in your best interest to try bodybuilding so that you use your strengths to your advantage on stage.

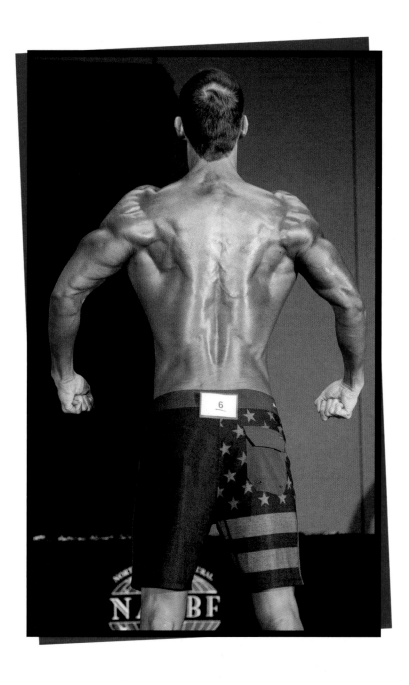

WOMEN'S DIVISIONS

Women have four divisions: bodybuilding, physique, figure, and bikini. Each division has a certain look based on muscularity, conditioning and muscular definition, and symmetry.

Women's Bodybuilding

Muscularity   The goal is simply to be as muscular as possible. Just as in men's bodybuilding, the more muscle, the better.

Conditioning and Muscular Definition   Conditioning in women's bodybuilding is the most extreme of all divisions, and the objective is to get as lean as possible. However, you should not pursue fat loss to the point where you sacrifice muscularity.

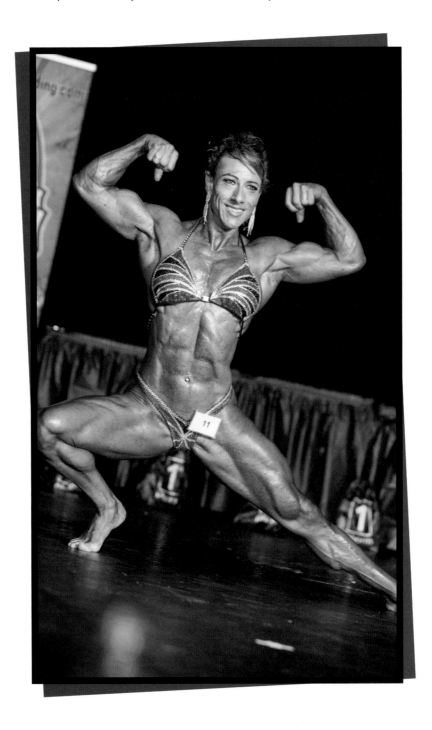

Symmetry   The criteria for muscular symmetry in women's bodybuilding are an even balance of development among all muscle groups. For structural symmetry, it is ideal to have wide-set shoulders, a small waist, and narrower hips.

Additional Considerations   The criteria for women's bodybuilding and men's bodybuilding are almost identical. The goal is to get as muscular and lean as your genetics allow. Women in the body-building division are not supposed to be judged on femininity, makeup, or hair, but we have seen these things become a factor at times. Give some consideration to makeup and hair; many judges will lump this in with overall stage presentation, even though they are not supposed to.

For this division, women do not wear heels. Typically, women's bodybuilding suits are one color and do not have rhinestones or sequins (although you should check the rules of the sanction you are competing in).

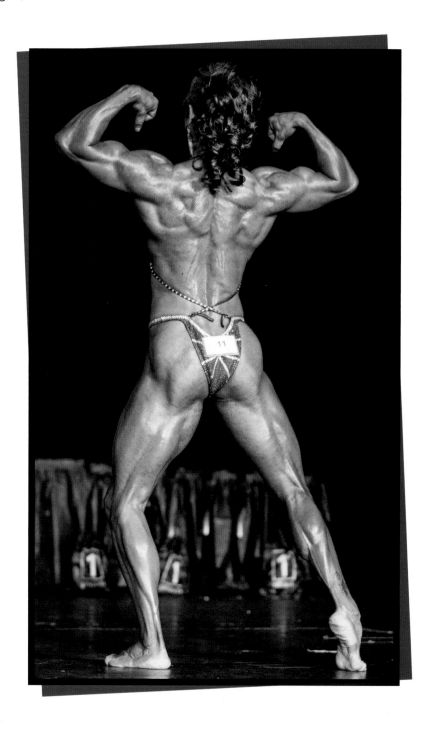

Women's Physique

Muscularity   Ideal muscularity for the women's divisions can be hard to determine. If women's bodybuilding aims for maximum muscularity, then women's physique would best be described as slightly less than that maximum. Even though the criteria for women's physique call for less muscularity than in the bodybuilding division, both authors find it rare for a drug-free female to achieve a look considered too muscular for this division. Most women have best results training for maximum muscularity.

Conditioning and Muscular Definition   Although the criteria for women's physique call for being slightly less lean than in the women's bodybuilding division, in real life, most competitors who place highly in women's physique achieve maximum conditioning. The goal should be to get as lean as you can.

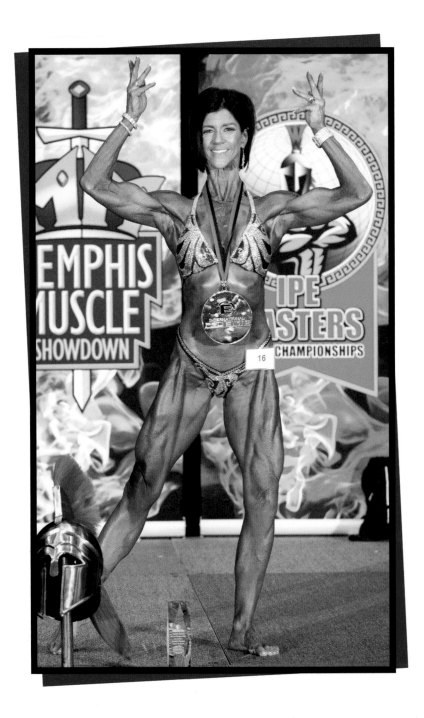

Symmetry   The criteria for muscular symmetry in women's physique are pretty much identical to those in the bodybuilding division. The goal is to have an even balance of development among all muscle groups. For structural symmetry, it is ideal to have wide-set shoulders, a small waist, and narrower hips.

Additional Considerations   Some sanctions require a rhinestoned suit and heels for this division, but some sanctions do not. Be sure to check with your sanction or promoter before the show so you know what they require. Typically, hair and makeup are considered part of the presentation portion for this division. This does not mean judges expect you to look like you are in a beauty contest, but choosing makeup and hair that is suited for you is important.

For the women's physique division, there is not a lot of difference between women's bodybuilding and women's physique. However, the posing is more feminine, and an overall physique deemed a bit more feminine will be judged more favorably here than in bodybuilding. This must be considered when deciding between the two divisions.

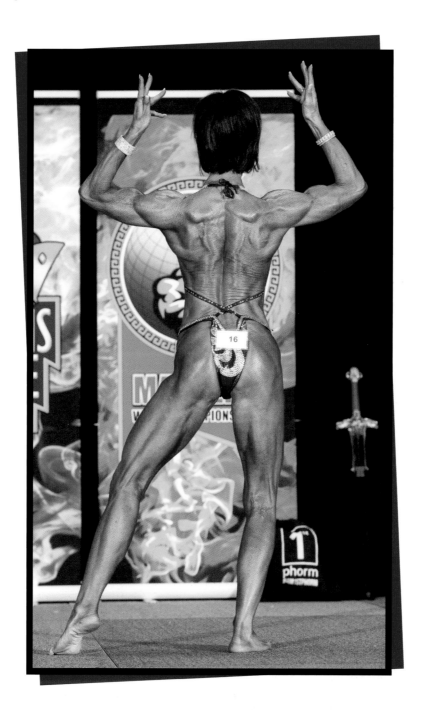

Figure

Muscularity   The muscularity requirement for the figure division is slightly below that of women's physique. In the drug-tested sanctions, there is not a lot of muscularity difference from the ideal women's physique competitor, but there is a slight difference. However, in untested competitions there is indeed a difference. If women's bodybuilding muscularity is described as maximum, then the ideal figure muscularity would be described as moderately high.

There are also differences between the amateur and pro levels, specifically in drug-tested competitions. In the amateur levels, judges look for a slightly lower level of muscularity, but on the drug-tested pro level, some women will have muscularity near a bodybuilding level.

Conditioning and Muscular Definition   In figure, the ideal conditioning can be a bit subjective. Aim for a look slightly softer than in the bodybuilding and physique divisions. The ideal look for figure shows separation between the muscle groups but does not have extremely striated muscularity. There should not be visible glute striations in the figure division.

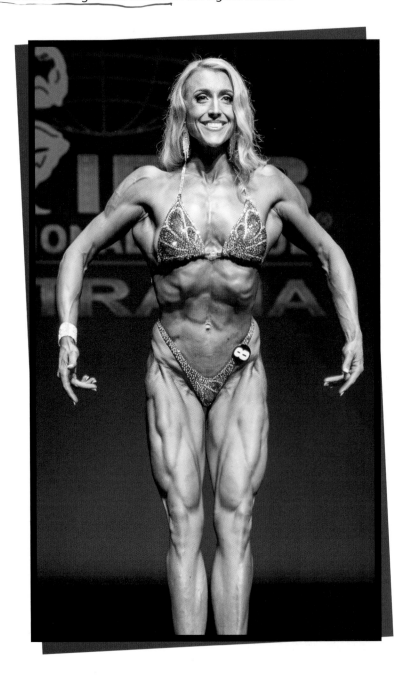

Symmetry   Structural symmetry in figure is even more important than in women's physique and bodybuilding because in those two divisions, there are many other ways to beat your opponent (such as getting leaner and having more poses to display muscularity). However, since there are only four poses in figure, having naturally wide shoulders and hips and a naturally narrow waist can be a powerful advantage. The typical feminine hourglass figure is desired in this division.

Muscular symmetry is similar to the other divisions in that you should strive for balance between all muscle groups, although figure favors greater muscularity in the shoulders.

Additional Considerations   In all sanctions, the figure division requires a rhinestoned suit and heels. Having professionally done makeup and hair is important because presentation is a bigger portion of the judging. This division is generally considered even more feminine than bodybuilding or physique—not that the authors (or most judges) are qualified to determine what is feminine and what is not. But most criteria state that competitors should display a muscular yet feminine physique.

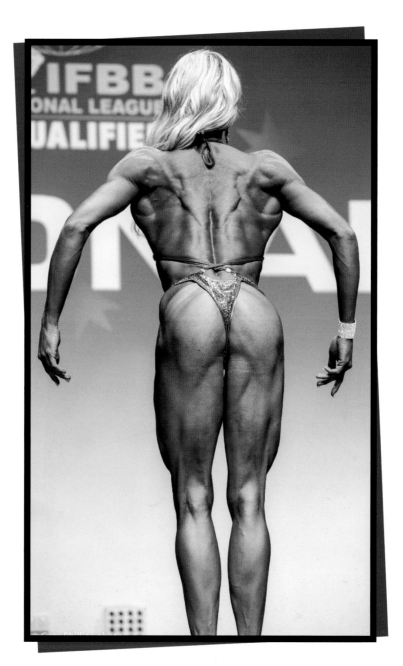

Bikini

Muscularity   Just as figure had a lower muscularity requirement than the previous two female divisions, bikini has an even lower requirement for muscle size. If figure muscularity is described as moderately high, then bikini muscularity would be described as moderate. Competitors in the bikini division should be fit but not necessarily muscular.

Conditioning and Muscular Definition   The bikini division also has the softest look of all the women's divisions. The precise amount of muscular definition that a bikini competitor should have is hotly debated. In fact, different sanctions often differ in their judging based on what they consider the ideal conditioning. This standard may even differ between shows within the same sanction depending on the judging panel. Generally, a bikini competitor should have visible abdominal muscles but not deep separation. It is ideal to have slight muscle separation in the shoulders and back but not striations.

A crucial factor in bikini conditioning is partially genetic. People hold fat in different places, meaning some people have an advantage in achieving ideal bikini conditioning. Typically, those with a naturally lean midsection will be favored because they can get a tight midsection without looking too hard or striated in other areas.

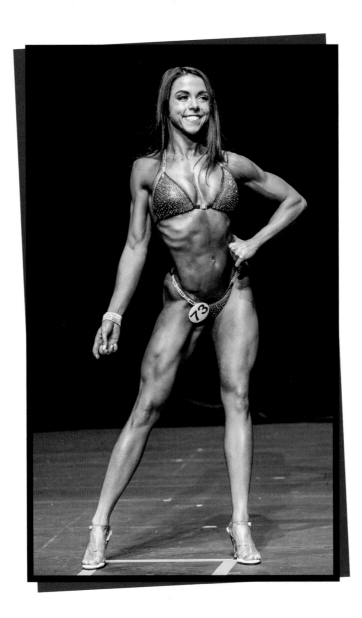

Symmetry   In bikini, just as in figure, structural symmetry is important. Whereas figure has four poses, in most sanctions bikini only has two poses: the front and back. Having a well-balanced structural look is crucial because you will not have many opportunities to overcome any structural deficiencies.

The glute and deltoid muscles are the two primary components of muscular symmetry for bikini. When structuring your training for a bikini competition, make these two areas a priority because judges look there. Balance training for the rest of the muscle groups accordingly.

For bikini, body fat symmetry plays a role in success. As mentioned earlier, natural body fat distribution varies. Some people store fat more evenly across the body, while others store fat in pockets. This normally does not matter in the other divisions because competitors need to get so lean that it will balance out with time. However, bikini requires a softer look, and the competitors carry more body fat than other divisions. Those with a more even body fat distribution fare better than those who tend to store fat in pockets.

Additional Considerations   Bikini competitors should have a rhinestoned or decorated suit, and the bikini division requires heels on stage. Just as in figure, makeup and hair are part of the presentation criteria, and competitors are expected to have a feminine appearance.

More so than any other division, bikini competitors are judged on presentation factors and less on physique. This means your smile, your walk, and general air of confidence can all be judged. This should also be considered when choosing which division to compete in.

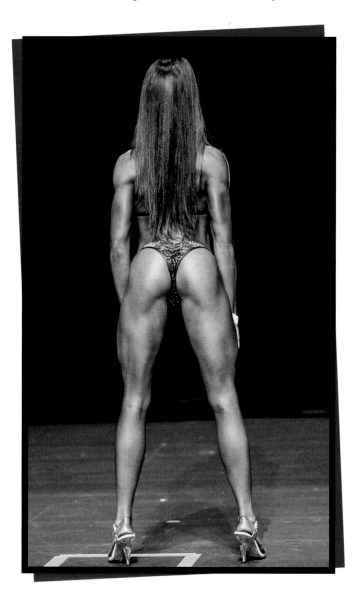

FAQ: Can a competitor compete in more than one division at a show?

Some shows allow competitors to compete in multiple divisions at the same show. However, the ideal look desired in each division differs. This means that what helps a competitor place highly in one division may hurt placing in another. Typically, it is difficult to place highly within multiple divisions at the same show; however, we have seen it happen.

FINAL WORD ON DIVISION CRITERIA

You may notice that the criteria descriptions seem rather vague and that there is no completely clear definition for each division. This is both the trouble with and the beauty of a subjective sport. There cannot be any absolute ideal for any division because different people have different preferences, bodies, and looks.

When choosing a division it is important to realize that, due to genetics, what looks best on one person may not look good on you. Understand that the precise look for each division is fluid. The look that the judges determine to be ideal can change from show to show based on the overall look of the lineup, and it can also change from year to year as trends change. Do not let the options overwhelm you; instead, train for the division of your choice and continue improving over time to meet the criteria.

FAQ: I feel like I may be able to compete in more than one division. How do I choose the best division for me?

Sometimes a competitor may fit in multiple divisions. In these situations, we recommend reviewing the previous physiques that have been successful at your target competitions to determine where your physique may fit best. In addition, if you are on the fence about which division to enter, consider the type of look you would like to present onstage when selecting a division.

CLASSES

Once you have an idea of which division you will compete in, the next decision is the class to compete in. Within each division, several different classes are typically offered. This is often a point of confusion for new competitors. Understand the differences between classes so that you enter the best classes for you at this point.

Classes Based on Age

There may be several classes at a given contest that are based on age. Although each show differs in which classes they offer, the following is a general guideline to classes based on age. Check with the show where you are competing for specific age guidelines.

Teen

The teen class is open to competitors 19 years old and younger. Some competitions may also offer multiple teen classes (under 17 years old, under 19 years old, and so on); however, most competitions offer only one teen class: for those 19 years old and younger.

Junior

Some competitions offer a junior class with a maximum age typically around 22 to 24 years. However, this class is not offered at many competitions.

Submasters

This class is open to individuals aged 35 to 39 years. It is offered at many competitions but not all.

Masters

Nearly all competitions have a masters division. This class is open to those aged 40 and over; however, in some divisions, the masters class may begin at age 35. Some competitions also offer a grand masters class of age 50 and over and an ultra-grand masters class for those older than 60.

Classes Based on Experience

Many competitions also offer classes based on experience or performance in previous competitions.

Debut and Beginner

Some competitions offer a debut class for individuals who have not previously stepped onstage. However, this is not offered at many competitions.

Novice

A novice class is for those who have not yet won a class or placed above a certain point in a larger class (usually the top three). Most individuals in this class are new to competing.

Open

This is the most competitive amateur class because it is open to all amateurs. Winners of each open class will compete for the overall title. If a competition is a pro qualifier, the open overall winner receives a pro card.

FAQ: Why are there multiple classes within the same show? For example, why are there three open men's bodybuilding classes?

When many competitors sign up for the same class within a division, the promoter may decide to split competitors into multiple classes. This helps to ensure that everyone has time to get a fair comparison to the other competitors onstage.

Bikini, figure, and men's physique classes are commonly split by height. However, bodybuilding classes may be split by height or weight, depending on the sanction. Sanctions such as the NPC, NGA, and INBF typically split bodybuilding classes by weight, while sanctions such as the NANBF and OCB typically split by height.

When there are multiple classes, the winners of each class are often compared in an overall. For example, if there are lightweight, middleweight, and heavyweight classes of open bodybuilding, the winners of each class will be compared against each other to determine the overall winner. If the competition is a pro qualifier, the overall winner receives a pro card.

Professional

This class is only offered to competitors who have won a pro card. You earn a pro card by winning an open overall title at a larger amateur competition (NPC national-level competition or designated drug-tested pro qualifier). Competitors in the pro class compete for prize money, but amateur classes do not award prize money.

FAQ: Can competitors make a living from prize money earned in professional competitions?

While competitors can win prize money in a professional bodybuilding competition, it is typically not enough to quit a day job, aside from a few top bodybuilders in the IFBB. Typical payouts for winning a professional drug-tested bodybuilding competition range from $500 to $1,000 for smaller competitions and up to $5,000 for larger competitions such as a world championship. Although IFBB competitions typically award larger monetary prizes than drug-tested professional competitions, it is still not enough for most competitors to make a living by competing. However, many professional bodybuilders are highly successful in their real-world jobs as well due to their work ethic.

Other Classes Offered

Some competitions have classes based on other factors or conditions not related to experience. To be sure you properly qualify for one of these classes, check with the show where you are competing for specific guidelines.

Classes Based on Profession

On occasion, classes may be offered based on the profession of the competitors. Common examples are a police and fire class or a military class.

Collegiate

Many competitions also offer a collegiate class for current college students. However, this class often has an age cap, so those considering the collegiate class should consult the show guidelines.

Transformation

Some competitions offer a transformation class for individuals who have made a large visual transformation to get onstage. These classes typically involve submitting a picture from a time before the competitor's fitness journey and comparing it to his or her current physique.

Classes for Individuals With Special Needs

Classes are often offered for individuals with special needs. This may include physical disabilities such as paralysis, cognitive impairments such as Down syndrome, and others. *Super cool*

FAQ: Can a competitor compete in more than one class at a show?

Most competitions allow you to compete in more than one class, provided you are qualified to enter each class. Typically, there is a crossover fee for entering more than one class. Consult the competitor information or contact the promoter for the specific show for details on crossing over between classes.

Criteria Defined

- **Muscularity** refers to how much muscle mass a competitor carries. The more muscle you build, the more muscular you are and the higher your level of muscularity. Some divisions call for high levels of muscularity, and others call for lower levels.

- **Conditioning** and **muscular definition** are essentially synonyms and refer to the absence of body fat. The leaner you are, the more conditioned you are and the more muscle definition you will be able to see. Being lean (having less body fat) ensures that your muscularity can properly show through. Divisions vary in their ideals for conditioning.

- **Muscular symmetry** refers to even development of all muscle groups. Some divisions call for a bit more development in certain areas, but in general the goal is evenness. **Structural symmetry** refers to how your body is put together: how wide your clavicles are set, how narrow your waist is, how long your arms are, and so on. Although muscular symmetry can be changed through training, structural symmetry cannot because it is dictated by genetics. However, certain structures may mean you are more suited to do well in one division over another.

Take-Home Points

- ▶ More divisions are offered at competitions than ever before, and the ideal look is different in each division. Understand the different standards for each division so you can choose the division that best suits your physique.

- ▶ Standards within a division may differ slightly from sanction to sanction or even between competitions within the same sanction. If possible, review the physiques that have been successful at your target competitions and pick a division based on where your physique will likely fit best.

- ▶ Classes at a competition are primarily based on a competitor's experience and age. Understand which classes you are qualified for so that you can enter the classes most appropriate for your physique at this point in your competitive career.

4

The Reality of Readiness

Prepping for a bodybuilding contest is hard! People look at their favorite competitors and think, "I want to look like that." The problem is that too few people stop to ask themselves what is required to make it to the stage successfully.

There is a difference between getting on a bodybuilding stage for fun and getting on a bodybuilding stage *at your very best*. In their zeal to compete, far too many people do not take the time to get themselves in a good spot, both mentally and physically, before contest prep. Let's look at what it takes to be ready to compete.

NEW COMPETITORS

The two most helpful things that someone new to the sport can do to foster success is to give the needed time to gain muscle and to attend shows to learn all the ins and outs of the sport.

Build a Foundation

It is not uncommon for people to discover weight training and immediately decide that they would like to compete. With no more than a few months of training, they announce to the world they are prepping for their first bodybuilding show. Then on show day, they are disheartened because they place poorly and wonder what happened.

This is because in a sport largely based around muscularity, they have given themselves almost no time to build the muscle required to compete. To build the needed muscularity, you must dedicate a significant amount of time to training hard and eating in a caloric surplus. Three years of training while eating plenty of calories is far different from three years of training primarily in a caloric deficit trying to lose fat. The former will result in far more muscle mass than the latter. Give yourself plenty of time to train, eat, and build new muscle.

Your genetics and the category in which you intend to compete dictate the time needed to build muscle. For example, those competing in the bikini division need less time than those competing in the bodybuilding division, just as those with naturally muscular physiques need less training time than those with naturally thin structures. It may not seem fair, but it is just the way it works. While there is no definitive rule, we have provided a general guide for how long you should train before you make your way to the competitive stage in table 4.1.

Table 4.1   Recommended Years of Serious Training Before Competing by Division

DIVISION	YEARS
Bikini	1-3
Figure	2-4
Men's physique	2-4
Women's physique	3-5
Classic physique	3-5
Women's bodybuilding	3-5
Men's bodybuilding	3-5

There are a couple of factors to keep in mind about these time frames. The first is that genetics largely dictate how long you need to train before you step on stage. As noted previously, some people have the genetic ability to build muscle more quickly and need less training time. Other people may have poor genetics for building muscle and require more time. Second, the time described in table 4.1 is needed *before* beginning contest prep and should be largely spent in a caloric surplus rather than dieting and trying to lose fat. Another factor to consider about these time frames is that this is typically the amount of time needed in order to be ready to compete adequately. If you are competing to win, you will probably require even more training time before stepping on stage.

Attend a Competition

Although attending a show before you prep is not an absolute necessity, it is probably a good idea because it gives you a clearer picture of what you are working toward, a sense of the contest rules, and an understanding of how a show is run. Consider this like doing your homework before a test. While you can still do well on the test if you have not done the homework, your chances of doing well are increased if you completed the assignment. Go to a show and see what it is like, and you will pick up some added motivation along the way.

To have a complete view of what happens on contest day, attend both the prejudging and the night show of a competition. However, if you are only able to attend for part of the day, we encourage new competitors to attend prejudging (the preliminary round of judging), where most judging occurs at a competition.

FAQ: As a new competitor attending a competition for the first time, is it important for me to attend a competition in the sanction in which I plan to compete?

Sanctions may run shows differently. Therefore, it would be a good idea to attend a show within the same sanction you plan to compete. This is especially important when looking at drug-tested versus untested competitions because the physiques onstage may be drastically different depending on your division. To get a more accurate representation of the physiques onstage at your competition, attend a drug-tested show if you plan to compete in a drug-tested competition or an untested show if you plan to compete in an untested competition.

EXPERIENCED COMPETITORS

For those who have gone through the contest prep process and competed, contest readiness is based on giving yourself enough time to recover from the last show and improve for the next show at a rate in line with your genetics, age, and experience.

How Long Since Your Last Show

Rushing into prep is a mistake that also plagues seasoned competitors. Often, after people finish a show, they experience one of two reactions: If they placed well and experienced a high from the sense of accomplishment, they cannot wait to get back on stage to get that feeling again. Or, if they placed poorly, they want to get back on stage as soon as possible to redeem themselves.

Both reactions lead to getting back on stage far too soon. Take time between shows because muscular growth takes time. This is especially true for drug-free competitors. If your goal is to get better from one show to the next (and that should be the goal for everyone), then you need to spend significant time eating in a caloric surplus and building muscle.

After a show, you must first recover from your contest prep before you can begin to make new progress. Research has shown that full recovery of testosterone, cortisol, metabolic rate, thyroid hormone, and muscle mass can take anywhere from two to six months (2, 3). It is unrealistic to think that a two-month off-season, for example, is enough to make significant progress between contest seasons.

Typical Progression Rate

The rate at which people can make visual improvements in their physiques varies significantly. Genetics, age, and training experience play a significant role in the rate of progression. Here are a few things to consider when deciding how much time you should take between shows.

Genetics

As noted previously, some people build muscle more quickly than others; this has been documented in scientific literature (1). Those who can build muscle quickly can usually take less time between shows and still make significant progress. If you take a long time to add muscle mass, take more time between shows to allow yourself time to improve.

Age

Natural levels of anabolic hormones and recovery rates are at their peaks during teens and early twenties. These are the prime growth years, and around age 25, there is a steady decline in growth potential. This means that younger people may need less time between shows to make significant progress. However, just because a younger person can make progress with less time between shows does not mean that he or she should compete more often. Both authors agree that if a competitor is truly dedicated to maximizing long-term potential, younger competitors should not waste their prime growth years spending a lot of time dieting for shows.

Training Experience

We have all seen people who are always dieting for a show yet, from year to year, seem to get bigger and more muscular. How is this possible? Does not this fly in the face of everything we discussed so far? In a situation like this, if you do a little digging, you often find that this person has been training less than five years. Most people see the most dramatic progression in the first five years of training. During this time, it is not uncommon to see people lose fat and build muscle at the same time even on very low calories. When they do eat enough calories, they can add size quickly. When someone competes often and still progresses, this is usually a short-lived effect. It may continue for a few years, but as training experience increases, the person sees progress slow down and may eventually regress without adequate time between shows. The longer you have been training, the longer you need between shows to make improvements.

There is no hard rule for how long you should take between shows, but a good range would be to take at least 16 to 36 months between shows to see significant visual improvement onstage for natural competitors. Those competitors using PEDs will require less time between shows since progress and recovery are accelerated by drug use. For most competitors using PEDs, 8 to 24 months between shows should allow enough time for visual progress to be made. Most of this time should be spent in an energy surplus.

FAQ: Would you ever recommend competing with less time between shows?

The 16- to 36-month range previously listed is how long we would recommend between contest seasons to see visual change. However, it is common to compete in multiple shows within the same contest season. We recommend choosing multiple shows within a one- or two-month period rather than dragging out the amount of time spent stage-lean. More information about how to handle competing in multiple shows can be found in chapter 12.

READINESS FOR CONTEST PREP

Regardless of whether you are new to the sport or have competed many times, everyone needs to have an effective mindset and enhance the ability to have an optimal metabolic capacity, manage any existing injuries, follow a plan, and withstand the financial and psychological impact of contest prep.

Acquiring an Effective Mindset

Developing an effective mindset comes naturally to some and through great hardship to others. When getting ready to start a contest prep, it is not uncommon to hear people say things like, "I'll accept nothing less than victory" or "Failure is not an option." When people say these things, they think they are showing others, and themselves, just how much they want this. However, as experienced coaches, we say that this type of talk is usually born out of desperation rather than determination, and to the untrained person, the two mindsets can seem eerily similar.

It is common for people to focus on the *goal* when it comes to bodybuilding. They focus on the show they want to win, they focus on wanting to add 20 pounds (9 kg) of muscle, or they focus on turning pro. While having goals is fine, the most effective mindset is one that places goals as the secondary focus and places the *process* as the primary focus. Focusing on your goal does absolutely nothing to help you achieve your goal. It is merely a distraction from what actually helps you achieve your goal, which is carrying out the process as effectively as possible and with as much effort as possible.

Let us put it another way. Assume that you are running a marathon. Your goal is to cross that finish line and prove to yourself that you can do it. It would make no sense to pull out binoculars every few feet to look at the finish line. It will not help you get there any faster, and you are likely going to slow yourself down. Instead of looking at the finish line, focus on the steps directly in front of you. Bodybuilding is no different. Your goal is clear: to win or place as high as you can. However, focusing on your goal isn't going to help you achieve your goal. Focusing on your process will do everything to help you achieve your goal.

Another aspect to consider is that you must develop the ability to move forward regardless of outcome. Often those who are goal-focused rather than process-focused struggle after the goal completion. They are much like a donkey chasing a carrot on a string. Once the carrot is removed or eaten, they are aimless. You cannot become so focused on winning your show that losing will make you fall into a depression. And you cannot become so focused on winning that if you do win, you feel as though you have nothing left to prove. The most effective competitors always know that each success and each failure is only temporary until the next success or failure. In the end, the most effective mind-set is one that focuses on the process, examines the results rather than dwelling on them, and moves forward with an improved process.

Finally, you must enjoy what you are doing. A process fueled by enjoyment will be easier to carry out than one fueled by a desperate need for approval. Find the things that you love about training, dieting, and posing. If you do that, the rest comes easily.

Optimizing Metabolic Capacity

It does not matter if you are a first-time competitor or have been competing for 20 years. Before beginning any contest prep, you must make sure your metabolic rate is at a peak. Optimizing metabolic capacity is simple. You need to spend time getting food intake as high as possible and cardio as low as possible while still maintaining a reasonable body fat percentage.

Try to think of metabolic capacity like a gas tank. Everything that you can do to create fat loss should be placed into this metaphorical **metabolic tank**. This means any amount of cardio that you can add and any calories that you can cut can be placed into the tank. If someone is eating plenty of food and doing little to no cardio, the tank is full because he or she has plenty of ways to create fat loss by adjusting calories and exercise. However, if someone is only eating 1,000 calories per day and already doing 45 minutes of cardio daily, it means his or her tank is empty because nothing can be added to the tank by doing more cardio or cutting more calories without detriment.

Beginning contest prep with an empty metabolic tank is like taking a car ride with an empty gas tank. Eventually, things stall more quickly than they normally would. Obviously, you can always create more fat loss by cutting more calories and adding more cardio. However, you eventually reach a point where going to such extremes will be a detriment. Fat loss will not be ideal, muscle mass will be lost, and recovery will be at an all-time low. Your body could rebel against you if you do not break mentally first. This commonly leads to a worse look on stage.

Make sure you take enough time to increase food and decrease cardio while sustaining a reasonable distance from stage-lean before starting contest prep. Fill up that metabolic tank before embarking on the journey of contest prep.

Managing Injuries

If you are a serious athlete, the odds are that you are dealing with at least one minor injury at any given time. Injuries happen when lifting heavy objects day in and day out for years on end. However, there is a significant difference between the little nagging injuries, muscle strains, or minor "tweaks" that happen from time to time and the more serious injuries that set training back significantly.

During contest prep, you will lose some muscle mass, and recovery will be reduced. If your training capacity is already hindered at the start of contest prep, this is not a good spot to begin. Recovery from the injury will be slow, and if muscle mass has been lost due to the injury, it may not come back during prep.

Make sure you let any significant injury heal before entering prep. Training capacity and muscle mass should both be at an all-time high before starting.

Sticking to a Plan

A successful contest prep should be so consistent that it is almost boring. Day in and day out, you must be able to stick to your nutrition plan, perform your training and cardio, get plenty of sleep, and then wake up the next day and do it all over again. If you are not mentally able to do this or are not able to do it due to life's circumstances, you should not start prepping for a show.

We often encounter people trying to start a contest prep even though they have a wedding in five weeks, must leave the country for work in seven weeks, have an anniversary trip planned in 10 weeks, and have several other events planned in between. This does not mean it is impossible to continue a prep through all these events and trips, but it is usually not a recipe for success. It is possible to go through all these types of circumstances and hit your plan 100 percent, but you need to honestly ask yourself whether you are mentally ready to do so. There is never a perfect time to compete, but some times are better than others.

Bearing the Financial Impact

An often-overlooked aspect of competing is that it is not cheap! In addition to regular food and gym membership costs, there are expenses for contest prep, a contest entry fee, a sanction fee, a drug-testing fee (if at a drug-tested competition), tanning products, at least one posing suit, and heels and jewelry (if in a division that uses them).

If a competitor has makeup and hair professionally done for show day or uses a spray tan service, those are added expenses. In addition, if the contest is out of town, travel and hotel costs can be significant. Further, many competitors today work with a contest prep coach. While doing so can be extremely beneficial, it is also an added expense. Lastly, if you compete in an additional class, there will be an extra fee.

An approximate summary of the expenses associated with contest prep and show day are listed in table 4.2. A competitor needs to be aware of and prepared for the expenses associated with competing before jumping into contest prep. The last thing you want is to get partway through your contest prep only to find out that you cannot actually compete due to financial reasons.

Table 4.2 Approximate Expenses for Contest Preparation and Show Day

Essential costs	
Contest entry fee	$100
Sanction fee	$100
Drug-testing fee (for a drug-tested contest)	$50
Self-tan tanning products and oil	$50
Posing suit	$50 (male), $300+ (female)
Heels (if in the bikini or figure division)	$50
Jewelry (if in the bikini or figure division)	$50
Optional costs	
Professional makeup	$50-$100
Professional hair	$50+ (hair styling), $100+ (extensions)
Spray tan service	$100-$150
Travel	$20+ (gas if driving), $300-$500+ (if flying), $30+/day (car rental, if needed)
Hotel	$100+/night
Contest prep coach	$150+/month
Additional class fee	$20-$40 per extra class

Handling the Psychological Impact

The final factor to consider before embarking on your journey to the stage is the psychological impact of the sport. Make no mistake about it: bodybuilding prep comes with a psychological toll. Many people do not talk about that once you have gone through contest prep, you may never look at your body, or food, in the same way again.

After a contest prep, you may no longer be able to have a meal without considering the impact that it will have on your physique. Even if you are not actively prepping for a show, and even if you have long since stopped competing in the sport, it may always be in the back of your mind. You become more keenly aware of the flaws in your physique. Although most people are critical of their own bodies, you will always hold yourself to a higher standard because you have seen yourself in stage condition. As a result, you will often find yourself judging your own body against your previous best.

Some people can balance all this, feel comfortable with it, and use it to make them better and happier. For others, it can absolutely break them. Do not enter this sport lightly. You need to ask yourself whether these trade-offs are worth it to you.

Finally, many people train and compete in bodybuilding because they want to improve their bodies. However, if you enter this sport because you hate your body or have negative relationships with food, this sport will not fix the problem. In fact, it will likely only exacerbate the issue. Contest prep is extreme and restrictive in nature. We push our minds and bodies to the limit, but after the show, we must work to regain some level of normalcy (at least a bodybuilder's sense of normalcy). The transition is difficult even for a person who has a completely healthy body image and relationship with food.

Before beginning contest prep, resolve issues you may have with food or your body image and make sure you are in a healthy spot mentally. Even still, it is a good idea to consider the long-term impact that competing will have on your life and your sense of balance.

PATIENCE AND TIME PAY OFF

Consider this chapter as your checklist to determine if you are truly ready to compete. Anybody can rush to the stage and receive a participation trophy. However, it takes something more to show patience and aim to truly bring your best. Not everyone has the willpower to be patient and wait until ready. Set yourself apart from the pack and be the one willing to put in the necessary time.

Take-Home Points

- ▶ A first-time competitor should build enough muscle base and attend a competition before competing.

- ▶ Experienced competitors should ensure they have a sufficient off-season before beginning the next contest prep. Generally, an off-season of at least 16 to 36 months is necessary to see significant visual progress. The exact amount of time needed for each competitor differs based on genetics, age, and training experience.

- ▶ To be successful regardless of competition experience, you need to have an effective mindset and an optimal metabolic capacity, manage any existing injuries, follow a plan, and withstand the financial and psychological impact of contest prep.

Show Selection and Timing: The Secrets of Preparation

There is nothing like the feeling of looking at the show schedule for the year and choosing the show or shows you will compete in. Then things start to feel like they have a purpose, and the reality of show day begins to loom. In the previous chapter, we covered everything that needs to be in place before you are truly ready to start contest prep. If you have met all the requirements, it is time to begin your journey to the stage! Where do you start?

On the surface, selecting a show may seem easy. Many simply pick a show located near where they live. But a show can make or break the success of your season, and you need to find the right one.

SELECTING THE RIGHT SHOW

In our coaching careers, we have seen nearly 90 percent of prospective clients select a show that will set them up for failure. That astronomically high number is because people do not realize the importance of this decision. Even if you make all the correct nutrition adjustments and are losing weight week after week, if you have not given yourself ample time to prep for your show, then you are doomed to fail before you even begin.

Historically, a competitor determines the length of prep by using a completely arbitrary process. For many years, 12 weeks was considered the standard length of a contest prep. When you decided to compete, it did not matter how much weight you needed to lose. You began prep at 12 weeks out, no matter what. As the bodybuilding community has started to realize the benefits of a slower prep, the standard prep length has become 15 to 20 weeks. Even this period may not be enough for many competitors.

There should not be a one-size-fits-all approach to prep length. We would not give everyone the same diet, so why would we give everyone the same length of prep? A proper prep length should be determined by your individual situation, not a "standard" number of weeks. There is a big difference between trying to lose 20 pounds (9 kg) in 20 weeks and losing 40 pounds (18 kg) in the same period. These situations require a different prep time length.

Let us look at it a different way and apply a similar situation to a squat goal. If two people have a goal of squatting 400 pounds (181 kg), and one of them can currently squat 390 pounds (177 kg) and the other can currently squat 185 pounds (84 kg), would you give them both five weeks to hit their goals? Absolutely not! This is like determining the length of contest prep; always remember that context is king.

FAQ: What is the best time for me to start contest prep?

There is no *best* time to start dieting for a competition. Many individuals who wait for the best time end up never competing because something always comes up in life. Similarly, many competitors (primarily male) are waiting to compete until they feel they are "big enough." However, these individuals often end up never stepping onstage.

Ultimately, some times in life are easier or harder than others to diet down for a show. There will likely always be something going on in your life that you must work around during contest prep. Life does not stop just because you are dieting for a competition. You should not be using contest prep as an excuse to not live your life.

APPROPRIATE RATE OF LOSS

The first thing you need to know about an ideal contest prep is that you should keep a steady but slow rate of fat loss. Research indicates you want to be in the range of losing 0.5 to 1 percent of body weight each week (8). This **rate of loss** (ROL)—the weight loss that you must maintain to be ready by show day—is fast enough to keep contest prep moving but slow enough to better retain muscle along the way.

Case study data from drug-free male competitors showed weekly losses of 0.5 percent of body weight (15) resulted in greater muscle retention than weekly losses of 0.7 percent (9) or 1.0 percent (12). This means it may be advisable to stick closer to a weekly loss of 0.5 percent of body weight, especially during the late phases of prep when an athlete is extremely lean and most susceptible to muscle loss.

If you are male, this means you want to target an average weekly loss of about 0.75 to 1.5 pounds (0.3-0.7 kg). Female competitors should shoot for a weekly loss of 0.5 to 1.25 pounds (0.2-0.6 kg) or less.

Although this is a slower ROL compared to the traditional 12-week prep approach, this is ideal for several reasons. Most notably, slower fat loss can do the following:

- ► Lead to more retained muscle mass (5, 6)
- ► Result in fewer negative repercussions on training performance and recovery (3, 13)
- ► Reduce or slow metabolic suppression (10)
- ► Create a more sustainable mental state

The faster the ROL, the higher the percentage of weight lost from muscle tissue and the more negative effects you will see in your training. Although this small effect may not be much of a concern when trying to drop a few pounds or kilograms, muscle loss becomes a greater concern the longer you diet and the leaner you become. When body fat stores are low, the body increasingly looks to conserve fat reserves by breaking down muscle tissue when it needs energy. The slower you take it, the less this will happen.

FAQ: Does my weight need to decrease to get stage-lean?

For a competitor to achieve stage-lean levels of body fat without the scale going down, muscle mass needs to be added at the same rate that body fat is lost. Since most competitors have 15 to 30 pounds (7-14 kg) of body fat (or more) to lose in the four to six or more months leading up to the competition, this means a similar amount of muscle mass simultaneously needs to be added during that time to keep the scale numbers from trending down.

Beginners on steroids have been shown to gain as much as 13 pounds (6 kg) of muscle mass in the first 10 weeks of weightlifting. However, drug-free males new to lifting only gained four or five pounds (1.8-2.3 kg) of lean mass in the same study (2). If a person is an experienced lifter (which he or she should be if dieting down for a contest), female, extremely lean, in an energy deficit, or any combination of these circumstances, the rate of muscle gain is significantly slower.

In addition, as a drug-free competitor becomes leaner, hormone changes detrimental to muscle growth occur (15). This results in lean mass loss, even in successful drug-free athletes (9, 15). Although this loss is not all muscle, at least some of it is due to a corresponding reduction in strength commonly observed during contest prep when a person is extremely lean.

Taken together, this data suggests that for nearly every trained drug-free athlete, weight will decrease to become stage-lean because it will not be possible to add muscle mass fast enough to offset the reduction in body fat. This is likely the case for athletes using drugs as well, but it depends on the type of drugs the individual is using and his or her history of drug use.

BENEFITS OF LONGER PREP TIME

With a slow target ROL, your contest prep time will be longer than the traditional 12-week prep. However, there are several benefits to a longer contest prep time.

Increased Muscle Retention

A longer contest prep allows a competitor to diet at a slower rate. As discussed previously, slow rates of loss are associated with increased muscle retention. This is because the means necessary to see a slower ROL are not as extreme as those necessary for the rapid loss typical of the old-school approach to contest prep.

Therefore, you can eat more food and do less cardio while still reaching your targeted loss because the rate is slower. That leads to better performance in the gym, better recovery, and more strength (and muscle) retention during contest prep. Muscle retention is key for prep in any division because you are judged on the amount of muscle you display on show day, not how much muscle was on your frame at the end of your off-season.

Leaner Physique

This one is self-explanatory. If you have more time to diet, you have more time to get leaner. Conditioning plays a large role in judging for all divisions and is one of the biggest reasons competitors place lower than they expect. By giving yourself more time to diet, you will be able to retain more muscle mass yet also have time to get lean enough for your division.

Refeeds and Diet Breaks

One big advantage of a longer contest prep time is that your prep does not have to be a sprint to the finish. With extra time, you can have days where calories are closer to or even slightly above maintenance.

A single day where calories are higher is often called a **refeed day** in bodybuilding circles. The extra calories on these days typically come from carbohydrate because carbohydrate over-feeding has a stronger effect on increasing hormones like thyroid and leptin than fat or protein overfeeding do (1, 14).

We will discuss what to do on a refeed day in more detail in chapter 6, but for now, understand that dieting slowly allows you to incorporate days where calories (and carbohydrates) are increased closer to maintenance caloric intake. The advantages are increased performance in a workout on the day of or the day after your refeed day due to increased glycogen stores. The largest benefit to a refeed day could be that it can give you a mental break from a calorie deficit, which helps you stick to your diet.

While refeeds are typically just one or two days with an increased intake, a diet break can range from one week to several weeks. During a diet break, calories are close to maintenance to essentially stop fat loss. We will also discuss diet breaks in more detail in chapter 6. Longer diet breaks have a greater effect on performance in the gym, hormone levels, and psychology than a single refeed day. In addition, diet breaks can have a more significant effect on metabolic adaptation during dieting than a single refeed day. In fact, preliminary studies on diet breaks have found that individuals who incorporate diet breaks saw no detrimental effect on weight loss (18) or even increased weight loss (4).

Although these concepts will be clearer after our discussion of how to implement both techniques in chapter 6, we hope you can appreciate that incorporating refeeds and diet breaks during contest prep can be beneficial. With a longer contest prep time, you can incorporate these higher-calorie days and still reach your target body composition.

Ready Early

Advocates of the 12-week prep approach usually mention not wanting to peak too early. While you should not be ready months in advance, being ready a few weeks early can be a benefit because you can start increasing food and tapering cardio as the show approaches. If this is done conservatively, it will not result in body fat gain and can lead to increased muscle glycogen stores. For each gram of glycogen stored, three to four grams of water is pulled into muscle (11). Visually, this means a fuller appearance, so the muscle looks larger and pushes out more against the skin. In addition, greater glycogen stores mean a better performance in the gym and aid muscle retention.

Being ready early can also allow you to do a mock peak week so you can adjust what you're doing to meet your goal. When using a more aggressive (and risky) peaking protocol, it is never a bad idea to test it out ahead of time rather than going in blind the final week, when it counts. We will discuss peaking protocols in chapter 10.

Reduced Stress

Bodybuilding contest prep is both physiologically and psychologically stressful. Dieting to extreme levels of body fat results in significant alterations to many hormones, menstrual cycles, and overall mood (7, 15, 16).

Despite those things, competing is something you should enjoy; it should enhance your life, not stress you out. Typically, if you enjoy the process, you will work harder and stay more consistent, and as a result, the process will go more smoothly. A longer prep also allows you to roll with the punches a bit more to keep stress levels in check.

DETERMINING NEEDED PREP TIME

When it comes to determining the appropriate length of a contest prep, ROL is everything! Here are the steps to work through to estimate the amount of time needed for contest prep.

Step 1: Measure Your Current Weight

This one is easy. Just get on a scale.

Step 2: Know Your Predicted Show Weight

This one is tricky, and you must be brutally honest with yourself. If you have competed before, then you should have an estimate to work with. If you are a first-time competitor, this will be hard. We find that most first-time competitors overestimate the ideal show weight by about 8 to 15 pounds (3-7 kg). You are better off aiming low and not needing to go there versus aiming high and scrambling to go lower later.

Step 3: Determine How Many Total Pounds to Lose

This is a simple equation to determine the number of pounds you must lose during contest prep. You take your current weight (CW) and subtract your predicted show weight (SW); the answer gives you your pounds to lose (PTL).

$$CW - SW = PTL$$

Step 4: Determine How Many PTL per Week

This is another simple equation that gives you your target ROL. You take the PTL determined in step 3 and divide by the number of weeks until the show (WTS). The answer is your needed ROL.

$$PTL \div WTS = ROL$$

The ideal ROL differs from person to person. The easier you lose fat, the higher ROL you should be able to easily maintain. While there is no hard rule for the ideal ROL, we recommend the following guidelines (higher ROLs are rare):

- ► 0.75 to 1.5 pounds (0.3-0.7 kg) per week for males
- ► 0.5 to 1.25 pounds (0.2-0.6 kg) per week for females

If your necessary ROL is higher than this, slow down and pick a later show. On the other hand, if your needed ROL is lower than this, you could pick up the pace.

FAQ: Do I need to select a show before starting contest prep?

You do not need to select a show at the start of contest prep. In fact, this can work to your benefit. By picking your show later in prep and basing the contest choice on your progress, you will ensure that you are stepping onstage truly ready.

To make this easier, we provide an example of how to determine ROL. Assume we have a male competitor who currently weighs 200 pounds (91 kg) with a targeted SW of 170 pounds (77 kg). He wants to do a show 25 weeks away. Now we enter this into our equations.

$$200 \text{ (CW)} - 170 \text{ (SW)} = 30 \text{ (PTL)}$$
$$30 \text{ (PTL)} \div 25 \text{ (WTS)} = 1.2 \text{ pounds (0.5 kg) per week}$$

Our bodybuilder is within the acceptable ROL for this show. He needs to maintain an ROL of 1.2 pounds (0.5 kg) per week to be ready in time for his competition.

$20 \div 25$

Now let us run through that same scenario with our bodybuilder as he considers a show 17 weeks away.

$$200 \text{ (CW)} - 170 \text{ (SW)} = 30 \text{ (PTL)}$$
$$30 \text{ (PTL)} \div 17 \text{ (WTS)} = 1.76 \text{ pounds (0.8 kg) per week}$$

As you can see, for our bodybuilder, a show 17 weeks away would be above the ideal ROL. While he could rush the process and indeed be at that weight by show day, he will likely be at less than his best by doing so. He would be better off picking a later show instead.

ROL during contest prep will not be linear. Metabolic adaptation occurs for several reasons during contest prep (17) and is described in more detail in later chapters. This results in **weight loss plateaus**—weeks when there is no loss at all.

For example, if you start prep with 20 pounds (9 kg) to lose in 20 weeks, you need to lose at an average rate of one pound (0.5 kg) per week. Based on our previous discussion, this is within an acceptable ROL for a male or female competitor.

Now, say that your prep starts off smooth, and you hit your target ROL over the first four weeks. You lose four pounds (2 kg), but then you hit your first plateau and lose nothing in week 5. Now you only have 15 weeks to lose 16 pounds (7 kg), which increases your target ROL slightly.

You make the necessary adjustments, and by 11 weeks out, you have 12 pounds (5 kg) to lose. However, something unexpected comes up the next week, and you gain one pound (0.5 kg). Maybe you get sick, maybe you get injured, or maybe you slip up and cheat on your diet. Regardless, these setbacks happen in real life so it is foolish to ignore them. Now you have 10 weeks to lose 13 pounds (6 kg), meaning you need to lose an average of 1.3 pounds (0.6 kg) each week until your show to be ready. For a female competitor, this ROL is just above the top end of the target range and will likely result in sacrificing muscle to be ready in time. In addition, by having such a tight timeline, a male or female competitor would not have time to do things like have a diet break or test out a peaking protocol ahead of time.

Always give yourself more time than you think is necessary. This allows you to take things as they come during prep and still get stage-lean without sacrificing excess muscle. One easy way to do this (if possible) is to base the show you do on when you are ready. Begin contest prep with several shows in mind. As you get closer to these shows, pick specific shows based on when you are ready. If prep goes extremely well and you are ready early, you can do shows at the earlier end of this range, but if things take longer than expected (which is often the case), you have other shows to fall back on. This ensures that you will not have to change your target ROL and that you will be at your best when you step onstage.

As you can see, choosing a show is not as simple as pointing to the calendar and picking a date. There are a lot of working parts that come together in finding the right show. This important decision can either lead you toward center stage or have you standing off to the side, wishing you had given yourself more time.

FAQ: Could I achieve stage-lean levels of body fat in less time than you recommend?

You could achieve stage-lean levels of body fat in less time than we recommend, and many competitors have stepped onstage with shorter preps. However, you most likely would not be stepping onstage at your best. A shorter prep would require a quicker target ROL. This would require less food, more cardio, or both to create a larger calorie deficit. The result would be lower-quality workouts and more muscle loss. Increased muscle loss during contest prep would also mean that your stage weight would be lower at the same body fat percentage than had you dieted at a slower rate.

Take-Home Points

▶ The ideal weekly ROL for muscle retention during contest prep is 0.5 to 1 percent of body weight, with lower ends of this range being preferred. As a rough starting point, males should lose 0.75 to 1.5 pounds (0.3-0.7 kg) a week while females should lose 0.5 to 1.25 pounds (0.2-0.6 kg) a week. This means that the traditional 12-week preps are not long enough for most competitors to get stage-lean.

▶ There are several benefits to a longer contest prep, including increased muscle retention, more time to get leaner, time for diet breaks, refeeds, ability to test a peaking protocol, and a less stressful prep overall.

▶ When determining the length of your contest prep, include extra weeks to account for plateaus and to give yourself time for things like diet breaks and to practice your peaking protocol.

▶ If possible, pick your show or shows based on when you are ready rather than targeting a specific show from the start of contest prep. This reduces stress and ensures that you are truly at your best when you step onstage.

Fueling Your Physique for Contest Preparation

When most people think about bodybuilding diets, a restrictive meal plan filled with nothing but dry chicken breast and broccoli eaten out of Tupperware containers comes to mind. Make no mistake about it: Nutrition is key to reaching stage-lean levels of body fat, and a competitor's diet will be far from a free-for-all. However, some nutrition practices commonly associated with the sport may not be necessary and, in some cases, may be detrimental to progress. This chapter outlines an effective nutrition approach for contest prep, including guidance on how to make nutrition adjustments during contest prep to maintain your target rate of fat loss and bring your best look to the stage every time!

ENERGY BALANCE

Before we dive into specific nutrition recommendations, it is important to understand the important concept of energy balance. **Energy balance** is the difference between your energy intake and energy expenditure. If you consume more calories than you expend, you gain weight, but if you consume fewer calories than you expend, you lose weight. This means that during contest prep, you need to be in an energy deficit to achieve your target ROL.

Energy Intake

On the surface, this may seem incredibly simple. Since humans cannot create their own energy from photosynthesis like plants do, energy intake only comes from the foods eaten. However, several vital details regarding energy intake can affect a competitor's results. For example, the **macronutrient** (protein, carbohydrate, and fat) composition of the diet may affect the type of weight gained or lost. Moreover, consuming adequate **micronutrition** (vitamins and minerals) is important for overall health. Competitors need to track intake accurately and eat foods they enjoy on a schedule that allows them to stay consistent. We will touch on factors associated with energy intake in this chapter.

Energy Expenditure

On the other side of the energy balance equation is energy expenditure. This seems simple as well. However, **total daily energy expenditure** is the sum of the **basal metabolic rate** (the number of calories required for basic bodily function), **thermic effect of food** (approximately 10 percent of calories consumed are used to digest and absorb food), exercise activity, and **nonexercise activity** (all the other movement a person does outside the gym during the day). We will discuss recommendations for exercise and nonexercise activity in chapter 7.

To complicate this side of the equation, many energy expenditure components are altered in response to both an energy deficit and weight loss, reducing total daily energy expenditure and resulting in a weight loss plateau. (For the science behind the reasons metabolism adapts during a diet, see references 30 and 49.) Knowing how to adjust when a weight loss plateau occurs during contest prep is the key to maintaining a target ROL, so this chapter covers how to adjust for these variables.

CALORIC INTAKE

Before diving into caloric intake for contest prep, we will review appropriate ROLs. Ultimately, caloric intake will be set to achieve a target ROL.

As discussed in chapter 5, one of the most common mistakes competitors make is not giving themselves enough time to diet for competition. This results in a contest prep where weight is lost too quickly (thereby sacrificing muscle mass), the competitor is not lean enough on show day, or both.

A review on natural bodybuilding contest prep recommended that competitors lose weight at an average 0.5 to 1 percent of body weight each week for optimal muscle mass retention (21). Looking closer at the case studies on natural athletes preparing for competition, those dieting at a ROL closer to 0.5 percent of body weight weekly (19, 39) lost a lower percentage of weight as lean mass than those dieting at a ROL of around 0.7 percent (24) and 1 percent (36) weekly, respectively. Although more research is needed on this topic, these studies—along with our observations in practice—suggest that slower ROLs are more optimal for muscle retention during contest prep.

This means that optimal ROLs for maximum muscle retention will likely be 0.5 to 1.25 pounds (0.2-0.6 kg) weekly for females and around 0.75 to 1.5 pounds (0.3-0.7 kg) weekly for males. To achieve the level of conditioning required to be competitive onstage, give yourself plenty of time for a longer, more gradual contest prep.

Determining Appropriate Caloric Intake

Once you have set aside enough time to diet for a competition, the next step is to determine how many calories to consume. Although there are many equations that exist to help calculate maintenance caloric intake, we find that many of them are inaccurate when applied to real-life situations and are rather unnecessary. To effectively and easily determine caloric intake, you must first know how many calories you are currently consuming and how your body is responding to your current intake. If you are currently tracking macronutrients or calories, this is easy because you already know. Even if you are following a meal plan, you can plug it into a nutrition tracking app to get a good idea of your current caloric intake.

However, if you do not know your current intake, track everything you eat or drink for at least one week. Some people start altering things once they begin tracking what they eat, and that can affect determining the appropriate number of calories needed. Continue to eat normally, and do not change your diet so you get an accurate picture of your current intake. Note how your weight is changing. For example, if your weight is increasing, you are above your current maintenance caloric intake, and if your weight is decreasing, you are below your current maintenance intake. If your weight has been holding relatively stable, this is your current maintenance caloric intake. It is simple.

Once you have an idea of your current maintenance intake, you need to reduce calories below this point to enter an energy deficit and achieve weight loss. No diet, nutrient, or food source is going to change this fact. Many fad diets, bodybuilding diets, and eating systems have tried to cheat this system, but the cold, hard truth remains: If you are not in a caloric deficit, you will not lose weight. Plain and simple.

The next step is to determine how much to reduce your intake to create an energy deficit. Many people think that since one pound (0.5 kg) of body fat is approximately 3,500 calories, a 500-calorie daily deficit is needed to lose one pound (0.5 kg) of body fat a week. It is a good starting point but in practice may not always be the case due to differences in metabolic adaptation. Some people require a larger reduction in caloric intake to see loss while others may be able to get away with a smaller reduction. This has led researchers to question the "3,500-calorie reduction equals one pound of weight loss" rule (48).

If you have given yourself adequate time to diet for a show, it is typically best to initially err on the side of a smaller deficit. From there, you can make small adjustments to caloric intake and achieve an appropriate ROL. Using the maximum intake possible means performance in the gym remains high, which will help you retain more muscle. In addition, this approach gives you room metabolically to make additional adjustments if or when plateaus occur along the way.

On the other hand, competitors pressed for time need to be more aggressive with initial calorie reduction to ensure they see losses and do not fall behind. If you are going to be aggressive, it is better to do so in the early stages of prep so that you can get ahead of the curve and therefore be less aggressive down the homestretch, when you are leaner and more susceptible to muscle loss. In either situation, it will still be important to adjust caloric intake to achieve the target ROL throughout contest prep.

Accuracy of Nutrition Tracking

Competing is an extreme goal, and extreme goals are rarely achieved without extreme effort and measures. It will require more effort, precision, and sacrifice than if your goal was less extreme. While this applies to many areas of contest prep, a competitor has little room for error when accurately tracking nutrition.

We mentioned that people tend to change their diets when tracking, but even when they do not, humans are notoriously bad at tracking caloric intake. In large nutrition surveys, average underreporting of calorie intake is as high as 70 percent in certain subgroups (29). This is a significant difference between estimated and true intake. Perhaps the most classic example of caloric underreporting is shown in a study published in the *New England Journal of Medicine* in the 1990s (28). In this study, researchers recruited middle-age overweight and obese women who claimed they were not losing weight on 1,200 calories or fewer daily. During the 14-day study, the women reported eating an average just over 1,000 calories daily, but when researchers measured their actual caloric intake, it was over 2,000 calories daily. This means that nothing was "abnormal" about these women, and the real reason they were not losing weight is because they were consuming nearly double the number of calories they had thought.

At this point, you probably think that you track your intake more accurately than most people, including those from the aforementioned studies. While that is probably true, underreporting even occurs in trained dietitians. Dietitians are better at estimating intake than nondietitians, but even trained dietitians have been found to underreport intake by over 200 calories daily on average (13).

Untracked calories commonly come from several sources. Many people do not count calories from fruits and vegetables; however, these are not "free" foods, and they do have a caloric value. There are often errors associated with weight versus volume measurements. For example, 1/4 cup of peanut butter measured in a measuring cup may not weigh 2 ounces, and the macronutrient values on a food label are based on weight measurements, not volume. We recommend measuring weight rather than volume for this reason. Similarly, people often give themselves too much leeway with measurements. For example, if that 1/4 cup of peanut butter was heaping, and you consider it "close enough" to 2 ounces, you may be consuming quite a few extra calories. Condiments, beverages, vitamins, supplements, and any other food or beverage with a caloric value can be a source of untracked calories.

It is critical to look for errors in your tracking to ensure that you are accurate during contest prep. As a rule, anything you eat or drink *must* be tracked.

FAQ: What do I do if I fall off my nutrition plan for a day?

Get back on track the next day! Often, competitors punish themselves by cutting food further or doing extra cardio. In most situations, this is not necessary and may even lead to bingeing and noncompliance down the road. However, if this day occurs too close to your show, you may need to push harder with less food and more cardio. Worst-case scenario, you may need to do a later competition.

Typically, when someone overeats of out physiological hunger, he or she may take a few extra bites here and there, but if you are having an all-out binge, there is often an emotional component. Think about what emotions you were feeling at the time of the binge and look for the emotional triggers so that you can better handle the stressor the next time it comes around rather than turning to food. If bingeing issues become regular, it will be best to put competing on hold and address underlying issues related to food before dieting down for a competition.

MACRONUTRIENTS

Macronutrients are the energy-containing components of food and are an important consideration as you determine what your diet will be. This is where you get your calories from. The three macronutrients are protein, carbohydrate, and fat.

Protein

Protein provides four calories per gram, and its role is to help repair and build muscle tissue. In addition, proteins are involved in many processes that support overall health, such as turnover of organ tissue, hormone production, antibody production, and transport of nutrients and hormones throughout the body. Therefore, adequate protein consumption is critical not only for maximizing physique-related goals but also for overall health.

Common Food Sources

Protein is comprised of a combination of 20 amino acids. Protein sources are classified as complete or incomplete based on their amino acid compositions. Sources that contain adequate amounts of all 20 amino acids are **complete proteins,** and those deficient in one or more amino acid are classified as **incomplete proteins**. In general, animal sources of protein are complete sources, and plant sources are incomplete sources. However, there are exceptions to this rule. For example, quinoa and soy are complete sources of protein from plants.

To prepare for a contest, a competitor must consume adequate amounts of all amino acids; therefore, vegetarians must mix complementary protein sources to prevent deficiencies. Foods high in protein include meat, fish, eggs, dairy, soy, some grains (e.g., quinoa), protein bars, and protein shakes.

Recommended Intake

The current recommended daily allowance (RDA) of protein is 0.36 grams of protein per pound of body weight per day. This may seem extremely low to readers used to consuming at least one gram of protein per pound of body weight per day. However, remember that the RDA is the amount of protein required to support tissue turnover in sedentary healthy adults. This is not necessarily the same amount required to optimize muscle repair and growth in a resistance-trained athlete. A study in resistance-trained young women found that those who consumed just over one gram of protein per pound of body weight per day gained significantly more muscle mass than those consuming just above the RDA (12). In addition, another study showed that the estimated average requirement for protein intake in young bodybuilders may be as high as one gram of protein per pound of body weight per day (6). These studies add to scientific literature that supports a protein intake higher than the RDA to maximize muscle growth in athletes.

There is growing evidence that protein requirements are even higher for someone in an energy deficit who is extremely lean and training hard. In fact, a peer-reviewed paper on nutrition for natural bodybuilding contest prep recommended a protein intake of 1 to 1.4 grams of protein per pound of lean body weight per day (21). Considering most competitors preparing for a contest have little body fat, this means that intakes over one gram of protein per pound of body weight per day may be optimal for muscle retention during contest prep. In addition, there is preliminary evidence that overfeeding protein in resistance-trained athletes may result in less body fat accumulation than carbohydrate and fat overfeeding (27). Therefore, a case could be made for even higher protein intakes.

Another benefit of high-protein diets is that they increase satiety during weight loss, which means they can help combat hunger during contest prep (52). In our own coaching careers, we have had great success prescribing protein intakes as high as 1.3 to 1.8 grams of protein per pound of body weight for lean bodybuilders. As we will see in the section about individuality, there are situations where this may not be necessary.

Regardless, during contest prep, a competitor has a limited number of calories available to distribute between the three macronutrients. As a result, overfeeding protein may limit carbohydrate or fat intake (or both), thereby potentially negatively affecting results.

We recommend starting with a protein intake of one gram of protein per pound of body weight a day (or slightly more) to maximize muscle retention. This approach gives a competitor enough remaining calories to consume adequate amounts of carbohydrate and fat. If you find you can maintain your target ROL on a higher caloric intake, increasing protein intake beyond one gram per pound may be beneficial, provided you are still consuming adequate carbohydrate and fat to support performance in the gym and hormone production. However, if you have a significant amount of body fat to lose, you may need to consume a protein intake lower than one gram per pound to also consume enough carbohydrate and fat while staying in an energy deficit.

Dietary Fat

Fat is used for several processes in the body, including making up a large portion of cell membranes and the myelin sheath around nerves, energy storage, body heat, and hormone production (which may be of most interest to physique athletes). Therefore, to combat hormone decline during contest prep, an adequate fat intake will be key.

Common Food Sources

Dietary fat contains nine calories per gram and is commonly classified based on its chemical structure. Saturated fatty acids do not contain double bonds, and unsaturated fatty acids contain double bonds. Unsaturated fatty acids can be further broken down into monounsaturated or polyunsaturated based on the number of double bonds. The chemical conformation of a double bond can classify a fatty acid as a trans fat.

Fats are often labeled as "good" or "bad" based on their effects on health. However, individual nutrient and health studies are often difficult because humans do not eat just one food or nutrient.

Consuming more unsaturated fat (20, 32) and less trans fat (14) appears to be beneficial for health. However, the data on saturated fat is less clear. Saturated fat was historically thought to cause cardiovascular disease; however, research suggests that saturated fat does not influence cardiovascular disease or mortality (14, 43). This area requires further study.

Fat is found in many foods, including nuts, seeds, oils, fatty fish (e.g., salmon), meat, egg yolks, and dairy.

Recommended Intake

A fat intake of 20 to 30 percent of daily calories has been recommended to support adequate hormone production for natural bodybuilders preparing for competition (21). Periods in which intake dips to 15 percent may be necessary to help spare carbohydrates and protein, but we recommend minimizing the time spent at extremely low fat intakes during contest prep to support adequate hormone production.

In addition, a person should consider how much of fat is truly needed even though it is an essential nutrient. When starting a contest prep, protein is important for muscle retention, carbohydrates are important for performance in the gym, and fat is essential for proper hormone production. However, if someone has a high caloric intake, a fat intake of 20 to 30 percent of total calories might be more than necessary. So in this case, it may be advisable to have fat intake at a lower percentage when calories are high and at a higher percentage when calories are low.

Fat intake should be set at a specific level to cover essential needs, and it should be kept around that point throughout the duration of prep. In most cases, carbohydrate intake should be the primary macronutrient that is decreased when caloric reductions are needed. For example, if a competitor is consuming 2,000 calories and 55 grams of fat each day, this would constitute about a 25 percent fat intake. However, if total calories are eventually dropped to 1,700 per day but daily fat intake remains at 55 grams, this would constitute an intake of about 29 percent. Despite the increase in percentage, we recommend keeping fat intake around a specific level as prep progresses.

However, it should be noted that at some point, dietary fat may need to be reduced to keep caloric intake at a place where the individual is still achieving the target ROL. As we will discuss in the section on individual differences, there is no one-size-fits-all macronutrient breakdown.

FAQ: Are high-protein diets safe?

At the time we wrote this book, there was no evidence that high protein intakes are detrimental to health in healthy individuals. In fact, a study in healthy resistance-trained males found that consuming 1.2 to 1.5 grams of protein per pound of body weight per day for an entire year produced no adverse effects on any marker of health measured (4). That study was extended to two years in a subset of subjects, and no detrimental effects were observed (3).

Existing data in scientific literature does not seem to reveal any harm in exceeding the current recommendations. However, it may be wise to use caution with extremely high protein intakes during contest prep because you may cut into the number of calories available to allocate to carbohydrate and fat while staying in a caloric deficit. By consuming inadequate carbohydrate or fat, you may see greater muscle loss and suboptimal progress. Therefore, the increased protein demands during contest prep need to be balanced with carbohydrate and fat while staying within your caloric allotment.

Carbohydrate

Carbohydrates are the primary fuel source used during resistance training and high-intensity, short-duration forms of cardio. In addition, carbohydrates are stored in muscle as glycogen, which is used for energy during workouts. Adequate carbohydrate consumption during contest prep can also help spare muscle and reduce amino acid degradation.

Common Food Sources

Carbohydrates contain four calories per gram and are commonly classified based on the number of sugars linked together in their chemical structures. Monosaccharides (glucose, fructose, and galactose) are individual sugar molecules, disaccharides (lactose, sucrose, and maltose) contain two sugar molecules linked together, oligosaccharides contain 3 to 9 sugar molecules, and polysaccharides contain 10 or more sugar molecules.

Common sources of carbohydrates include grains, fruit, vegetables, legumes, dairy, and added sugars (such as table sugar and honey).

FAQ: Should I be concerned about sugar intake during contest prep?

There is no evidence that sugar consumption affects fat loss if macronutrient requirements are met each day. Diets high in fructose (the sugar found in fruit) have not been shown to affect weight loss compared to low-fructose diets (7). Similarly, diets high in dairy (lactose) have not been shown to inhibit fat loss (1).

However, foods high in added sugars are typically lower volume and higher calorie. Consuming a lot of calories from added sugar may lead to increased hunger due to a low food volume. In addition, many foods high in added sugars are micronutrient poor; therefore, we recommend consuming at least 80 to 90 percent of food from nutrient-dense foods to meet micronutrient needs.

For competitors with a low carbohydrate intake (i.e., 100-150 g per day or less), it may be advisable to limit fruit to one serving a day. This has nothing to do with fruit's effect on fat loss; however, fructose from fruit is primarily stored in the liver as glycogen, whereas glucose can be made into muscle glycogen. A diet high in fructose with a low carbohydrate intake may lead to further muscle glycogen depletion and a reduced performance in the gym. Therefore, it may be in your best interest to limit fruit intake to a certain extent if your carbohydrate intake is low.

Recommended Intake

A review of nutrition recommendations for bodybuilding contest prep suggests that carbohydrate consumption should make up the remainder of your caloric allotment once protein and fat are accounted for (21). In practice, we feel this may be a good starting point for most.

For example, if a 180-pound (82 kg) male is consuming 2,200 calories per day, he will first want to ensure he is consuming at least one gram of protein per pound of body weight; preferably even somewhat higher if he has the caloric allotment to do so. In this example, we will set his protein at 220 grams daily. He wants to keep fat in the 20 to 30 percent range to support hormone production, so he sets fat at 55 grams daily. This leaves 825 calories for carbohydrates, which are set at about 205 grams daily. Altogether, our competitor's starting daily macronutrient intake is 220 grams of protein, 205 grams of carbohydrates, and 55 grams of fat. Although individual needs may differ, this would likely be a good starting point for most male competitors.

INDIVIDUAL DIFFERENCES IN MACRONUTRIENT NEEDS

While it is easy to advise everyone to get into a caloric deficit and let nature take its course, things are not always that simple. Anyone who has been in bodybuilding for a significant amount of time notices that people react to diets differently. It did not take us long in our coaching careers to realize that if we gave a similar diet to two individuals who are the same height and weight, there would be two entirely different outcomes.

Figuring out individual diet differences comes from experience and trial and error. However, over the years, we have noted a few recurring commonalities. Let us look at several trends we have observed in our combined 30-plus years in the sport.

Gender

A good place to start with individuality is the difference between men and women. Women simply burn fewer calories at rest than men do. Research has shown that women's metabolic rates tend to be about 5 to 10 percent lower than men's metabolic rates (15). While this may not seem like a large difference, the slower metabolic rate per pound combined with lower overall body weight means many women require much lower caloric intakes. When you consider that it is normal for metabolic rate to slow during a contest prep, this can lead to some very low caloric intakes by the end of prep. This is completely normal.

It may be harder for most women to lose weight, but we have noticed that female competitors tend to retain more muscle mass during contest prep. While we are not entirely sure why, we hypothesize that this has to do with the fact that women's muscle mass is not as dependent on testosterone. During contest prep, men who are not using drugs see significant drops in testosterone, which can cause loss of lean tissue (39). However, drug-free women have such low testosterone levels to begin with that they will not see these losses during a contest prep. Therefore, women can dig harder with their diets and cardio than males and will not lose as much muscle. Because women require fewer calories, we find that they can respond better to lower protein intakes than men do. If protein is set too high, it will be hard to get total daily caloric intake as low as it needs to be for fat loss.

Race

There is not a lot of talk about racial differences for diet and bodybuilding, most likely because it is a sensitive subject. However, when you look at it from a practical standpoint, if differences in environment over time have resulted in differences in physical traits, it makes perfect sense that environment may affect metabolism over time as well. In our experience, most African American and Hispanic competitors tolerate a diet lower in carbohydrates and higher in protein and fat. This is likely due to higher rates of insulin resistance within these racial groups (18). To go along with reduced insulin sensitivity, African Americans in general tend to have lower resting metabolic rates than Caucasians (46). When you combine these factors, it can seem more difficult for African Americans to lose fat than it is for Caucasians.

Although it may be harder for African American competitors to get stage-lean, our experience has shown us that, much like we just discussed with female competitors, many African American competitors can maintain a higher level of muscle mass while reaching very low body fat levels. With this knowledge, if total caloric intake needs to get very low, protein intake should not be set too high; otherwise fat loss might be slowed.

History

Last, but certainly not least, you can learn a lot about individuality based on someone's history. As coaches, we know gathering a competitor's history is part of learning about the person as an individual. If someone has typically had a hard time losing weight, it is likely he or she will also have a harder time in the future. In our experience, those with a history of "hard case" fat loss respond better to plans lower in carbohydrates and higher in protein.

Macronutrient Examples for Men

When we look at primary individual differences, we can lay out a few examples of how differing diets may be set up to meet specific needs. Let us begin with a 180-pound (82 kg) male Caucasian competitor who has an average metabolic rate and a caloric intake of 2,200 calories. In our previous example in the Recommended Intake section, we set it up as follows:

- ▶ Protein: 220 grams
- ▶ Carbohydrates: 205 grams
- ▶ Dietary fat: 55 grams

An example of how this 180-pound (82 kg) Caucasian competitor may set up a daily meal plan to hit these macronutrient targets can be found in table 6.1. However, this is only one of millions of ways to set up a daily meal plan to hit these macronutrient totals. Your daily meal plan will differ from this based on your macronutrient needs, schedule, and food preferences.

With this 2,200-calorie intake example, if this competitor was a 180-pound (82 kg) African American competitor, we have had great success adjusting this macronutrient ratio to look something more like this:

- ▶ Protein: 250 grams
- ▶ Carbohydrates: 140 grams
- ▶ Dietary fat: 70 grams

Table 6.2 provides a sample meal plan of how this 180-pound (82 kg) African American male may meet his daily macronutrient allotment.

Note that these meal plans are only meant to be an example and likely are not best for you. Your specific meal plan will differ from tables 6.1 and 6.2 based on your macronutrient requirements, schedule, and food preferences.

FAQ: What is the best way to accurately measure my food?

Measuring cup and spoon sizes are variable and not always standardized. Further error is introduced based on the degree a measurement is heaped. Also, there can be large variations between brands. Although these deviations may not seem significant, inaccurate measurements made multiple times a day will add up and contribute to caloric over- or underreporting. The best approach is to refer to the nutrition label of each specific food and use a scale to weigh each item separately.

Table 6.1 Sample Meal Plan A

FOOD	AMOUNT* (UNCOOKED)	PROTEIN (GRAMS)	CARBOHYDRATE (GRAMS)	DIETARY FAT (GRAMS)
Meal 1				
Oatmeal (old-fashioned)	20 g (1/4 cup)	2.5	13.5	1.5
Egg whites	300 g (≈10 whites)	33	2	0
Low-fat cheese	28 g (1 oz slice)	7	0.5	2
Salsa	28 g (1 Tbsp)	0	2	0
Blueberries	100 g (1/2 cup)	1	14.5	0
Meal 2				
Low-fat cottage cheese	150 g (2/3 cup)	18	4.5	2
Mixed nuts	28 g (1/4 cup)	5	6	15
Banana	100 g (1 medium)	1	23	0
Meal 3 (preworkout)				
Chicken breast (meat only)	200 g (1 cup chopped)	45	0	5
Brown rice (long grain)	75 g (≈1/3 cup)	5.5	57	2.5
Broccoli	200 g (2 cups)	5.5	13	1
Postworkout				
Whey protein powder (shake)	40 g (≈1-2 scoops)	27	7	3
Meal 4				
Tilapia	150 g (≈5 oz)	30	0	3
Sweet potato	150 g (≈6 in. long)	2.5	30	0
Iceberg lettuce	100 g (2 cups)	1	3	0
Light salad dressing (vinaigrette)	28 g (1 Tbsp)	0	1	2
Meal 5				
Lean steak	150 g (≈5 oz)	33	0	12
Red bell pepper (chopped)	100 g (1/2 cup)	1	6	0
Low-fat chocolate ice cream	60 g (≈1/2 cup)	2	20	4
TOTALS				
Total		220	203	53
Goal		220	205	55

*The amounts for customary units in parentheses are approximations; for accuracy, we recommend using metric weight. See the previous FAQ for more information.

Table 6.2 Sample Meal Plan B

FOOD	AMOUNT* (UNCOOKED)	PROTEIN (GRAMS)	CARBOHYDRATE (GRAMS)	DIETARY FAT (GRAMS)
Meal 1				
Egg whites	400 g (≈13 whites)	44	3	0
Low-fat cheese	28 g (1 oz slice)	7	0.5	2
Salsa	28 g (1 Tbsp)	0	2	0
Blueberries	100 g (1/2 cup)	1	14.5	0
Avocado	100 g (1/2 of a whole minus pit)	2	9	15
Meal 2				
Low-fat cottage cheese	150 g (2/3 cup)	18	4.5	2
Mixed nuts	28 g (1/4 cup)	5	6	15
Tuna (in water) packet	74 g (1 packet)	17	0	1
Meal 3 (preworkout)				
Chicken breast (meat only)	200 g (1 cup chopped)	45	0	5
Brown rice (long grain)	75 g (≈1/3 cup)	5.5	57	2.5
Broccoli	200 g (2 cups)	5.5	13	1
Postworkout				
Whey protein powder (shake)	40 g (≈1-2 scoops)	27	7	3
Meal 4				
Tilapia	175 g (6 oz)	35	0	3
Sweet potato	60 g (1/2 of whole ≈5 in. long)	1	12	0
Iceberg lettuce	100 g (2 cups)	1	3	0
Light salad dressing (vinaigrette)	28 g (1 Tbsp)	0	1	2
Meal 5				
Lean steak	150 g (≈5 oz)	33	0	12
Red bell pepper (chopped)	100 g (1/2 cup)	1	6	0
Almond butter (unsalted)	10 g (2 tsp)	2	2	6
TOTALS				
Total		250	140.5	69.5
Goal		250	140	70

*The amounts for customary units in parentheses are approximations; for accuracy, we recommend using metric weight. See the FAQ for more information.

Macronutrient Examples for Women

In our previous example, we saw male competitors with caloric intakes set at about 12.25 calories per pound of body weight. Protein intakes were set at about 1.2 grams per pound of body weight (Sample Meal Plan A) and about 1.4 grams per pound of body weight (Sample Meal Plan B). Let us see how this might work with a 115-pound (52 kg) female competitor.

Since women have up to a 10 percent lower metabolic rate, we need to adjust this caloric intake to about 11 calories per pound of body weight. This means our female competitor needs roughly 1,265 calories. Let us see how we may set that up for this female Caucasian competitor:

- ► Protein: 125 grams
- ► Carbohydrates: 101.25 grams
- ► Dietary fat: 40 grams

Notice that our protein intake is set slightly lower for this female competitor at about 1.1 grams per pound of body weight. This is to account for the lower total caloric intake needed. Now let us look at the plan for a 115-pound (52 kg) African American female competitor consuming 1,265 calories daily:

- ► Protein: 138 grams
- ► Carbohydrates: 70.25 grams
- ► Dietary fat: 50 grams

In this instance, the changes are not substantial, but it would be much more likely to produce consistent results for an African American competitor. On a side note, once daily carbohydrate intake drops below 100 grams, we recommend that at least 40 to 60 percent of carbohydrate intake come from a variety of vegetables. This not only ensures nutritional needs are met but also helps with satiety.

While these examples only scratch the surface of the nearly infinite adjustments that can be made to account for individuality, they show how differing macronutrient ratios can be set up to help various populations. There are no hard rules. Although one population may be "more likely" to have specific needs, there are always exceptions. For this reason, we recommend looking at your individual needs and history as the primary indicators for how to set up your macronutrient ratios.

FIBER

Fiber is a carbohydrate not digested by human enzymes and is instead fermented by bacteria in the large intestine. There are a number of benefits of high-fiber diets (reviewed by (2)). The most notable for bodybuilders is that fiber increases satiety. Therefore, consuming a high-fiber diet makes you feel fuller than if your diet was low in fiber. Anyone who has been stage-lean will tell you that managing hunger and taking the edge off when consuming a lower caloric intake can go a long way toward increased adherence and success during contest prep.

Fermentation of fiber in the large intestine produces many byproducts, including short-chain fatty acids, which are absorbed by our bodies and used for energy. Therefore, fiber has a caloric value estimated as 1.5 to 2.5 calories per gram, depending on the composition of the fiber source. This is less than carbohydrates, which contain 4 calories per gram. However, to avoid confusion, count fiber along with other carbohydrates consumed and aim to have a consistently high fiber intake.

The Institute of Medicine recommends that adults consume at least 14 grams of fiber for every 1,000 calories consumed. This means that someone consuming 2,500 calories daily during contest prep should aim to get at least 35 grams of fiber daily. This level of fiber intake may not be possible when carbohydrate intake is low during contest prep. In this situation, it may be more practical to aim for at least 10 grams per 1,000 calories consumed.

It is common for fiber intake to increase during contest prep as a competitor consumes more high-volume, low-calorie foods to combat hunger. However, high fiber intakes can cause gastrointestinal (GI) distress. If you notice GI symptoms from consuming high amounts of fiber, reduce fiber intake to a better tolerated level.

VITAMINS AND MINERALS

Bodybuilders have historically eliminated several foods or even entire food groups when preparing for competition. Older bodybuilder case studies from the 1980s and 1990s reveal that it was common to eliminate fruit, dairy, sugar, egg yolks, and even red meat due to the fear that these foods would interfere with fat loss (22, 26, 47). As a result, it was also common for these competitors to be deficient in many vitamins and minerals, including calcium since complete elimination of dairy was part of the normal approach (22, 25, 26, 40).

There is no need to eliminate any food, nutrient, or food group during contest prep unless you have a diagnosed medical reason to do so. If anything, the deficiencies caused by this approach may negatively affect results. No food or food group will prevent weight loss. When individuals are in an energy deficit, they can literally eat anything they want and still lose weight, provided they remain in an energy deficit.

A study comparing the acute effects of a meal consisting of a Big Mac, fries, and a root beer from McDonald's to a homemade organic burger meal in which macronutrient intake was matched revealed no difference in insulin, glucose, free-fatty acids, blood lipids, or hunger hormones (9). In addition, several interesting case studies have been done to challenge the claim that food source matters more than energy balance for weight loss. John Cisna, a high school science teacher, lost a significant amount of weight only eating food from McDonald's because he was in a caloric deficit and exercising.

Dr. Mark Haub, a nutrition professor at Kansas State University, consumed a convenience-store diet consisting primarily of foods such as Twinkies. Dr. Haub lost a significant amount of weight because he was in a caloric deficit daily. Beyond these examples, thousands of bodybuilders get stage-lean every year without eliminating any food or food group. Although these studies have not been published in peer-reviewed journals or undergone the scrutiny of the peer-review process, they clearly show that energy balance drives weight loss, not food source.

Before you make McDonald's and Twinkies the staples of your next contest prep diet, there are a few things you need to keep in mind. The first is that you are still a human being, which means you have vitamin and mineral requirements that need to be met. In addition, when you are dieting, hunger will increase. Consuming one Twinkie to get 30 grams of carbohydrate is not going to satisfy you as much as consuming about two and a half cups of steamed broccoli to get 30 grams of carbohydrate. Therefore, in the interest of performance in the gym, muscle retention, dietary adherence, and overall health, consume a variety of foods from all food groups to meet your macronutrient needs. Also, aim for multiple colors in your fruits and vegetables to consume a variety of micronutrients.

Again, unless you have a diagnosed medical condition that requires you to eliminate a food or food group (e.g., lactose intolerance or celiac disease), there is no reason to eliminate anything if your macronutrient needs are being met consistently.

Some individuals may find that it is easy to have a different meal plan each day during contest prep, and others may find preparing their meals for the week ahead of time to eat the same meal plan daily works best to stay consistent. For those eating the same meal plan daily, it may be in your best interest to rotate in different foods each week. For example, have broccoli as a vegetable one week, have carrots instead the next week.

It may also be helpful to incorporate a combination of nutrient-dense food sources with other foods you want to eat. A good way to do this is to use an 80/20 or 90/10 approach, where you are consuming most of the food (at least 80%-90%) from nutrient-dense sources with other things you want in moderation (e.g., a serving of ice cream). However, as caloric intake is reduced, and you get closer to stage-lean, this ratio may start looking more like 95/5, 99/1 or even 100/0 because nutrient-dense whole foods are often more filling and can help keep hunger levels in check. Ultimately, the approach that allows you to meet your macro- and micronutrient needs while adhering to your plan daily is the approach that works best for you.

FAQ: Can I have artificial sweeteners during contest prep?

Artificial sweeteners are sugar substitutes that provide a sweet flavor with a lower caloric value than sugar. Research has shown that artificial sweeteners in amounts typically consumed by humans is safe (31). However, not all artificial sweeteners are calorie-free. Therefore, account for any calories into your daily allotment. If calories are accounted for, there is no evidence that artificial sweeteners affect fat loss (37).

It is common for competitors to consume an increasing amount of artificial sweeteners throughout contest prep to fight hunger. However, large amounts of artificial sweeteners (or sugar alcohols) can cause GI distress. If you experience GI distress from using artificial sweeteners, reduce how much you consume.

MEAL FREQUENCY

Bodybuilders have historically eaten more frequent, smaller meals daily. In fact, previous case studies on bodybuilders preparing for competition have reported as many as 10 meals a day (47). On the other extreme, intermittent fasting has gained popularity in the fitness community. Individuals using this approach consume food within a given time each day. Anecdotally, competitors have stepped onstage claiming success using both approaches; however, what does the scientific literature say?

Numerous studies on meal frequency and weight loss have not observed a difference in weight loss when daily calories are matched (11). Moreover, intermittent fasting has not been shown to be superior to more traditional meal patterns (42). Therefore, it does not appear that the number of meals consumed throughout the day affects weight loss if calorie intake is low enough to induce weight loss. From an applied standpoint, this means your meal frequency should be based on your schedule, preferences, and what allows you to stay consistent with your macronutrient intake each day.

However, scientific literature about meal frequency mostly reports studies done for overweight and obese individuals during weight loss interventions. This is a significantly different population than a bodybuilder dieting down to an extremely lean body composition. Bodybuilders need to also be highly concerned with muscle retention, not just weight loss.

PROTEIN TIMING

Consumption of a meal containing protein stimulates **muscle protein synthesis** (MPS), the rate at which new proteins are created in muscle tissue to repair and build tissue. However, the increase in MPS is short-lived (8). Therefore, bodybuilders have historically believed that more meals are better when it comes to keeping MPS elevated. However, there is evidence that if meals are spaced too closely together, the second meal may not have the same increase in MPS as the first (8). As a result, a paper on nutrition guidelines for bodybuilding contest prep recommended a more moderate meal frequency of three to six protein-containing meals daily to optimize muscle repair and growth (21). We agree that this would be a good starting point for most competitors.

There is also evidence that certain times may be more critical for protein (meal) consumption. Bodybuilders have notoriously consumed protein shakes immediately postworkout so that they did not miss out on the "anabolic window of opportunity." This is the time where MPS increases due to the combination of exercise and nutrition. However, research has shown that this window lasts at least 24 hours, with the greatest benefits shown within the first three hours after exercise (33). Therefore, we recommend consuming a meal containing protein within one or two hours postworkout.

A meta-analysis looking specifically at consumption of postworkout protein shakes failed to find a statistically significant difference in muscle size or strength gains when daily total protein intake was matched (41). However, there was a small trend toward favorable outcomes with postworkout protein shake consumption. For a bodybuilder looking for any possible small advantage, this may be enough to warrant consuming a protein shake after working out. There would not be any negatives if the shake protein content fits into your daily macronutrient numbers.

There is evidence that consuming protein before bed may have beneficial effects on muscle repair and growth (34). Therefore, we recommend consuming a meal containing protein immediately before going to bed. Although it is only anecdotal evidence, we have also found that consuming a larger meal before going to bed may help improve the quality of sleep for some competitors, especially when they reach extremes in body composition.

CARBOHYDRATE TIMING

Maintaining strength in the gym is key to holding on to muscle mass throughout contest prep. The primary fuel source used during resistance exercise is carbohydrate. Much of this carbohydrate comes from muscle **glycogen** (the storage form of carbohydrate in muscle). Studies have shown that lifting weights in a glycogen-depleted state reduces strength and increases fatigue compared to preworkout carbohydrate consumption (16). Therefore, a high-carbohydrate meal one to three hours preworkout may increase performance.

In practice, the exact number of carbohydrates consumed in this meal may differ between individuals. Some have improved performance in the gym after a large, high-carbohydrate meal, whereas others may feel like they want to take a nap after the same meal. For those in the latter group, it is best to adjust preworkout carbohydrate intake based on individual tolerance and performance.

Carbohydrate consumption during and after a workout has widely been studied in aerobic endurance athletes, where fast-digesting carbohydrates have been shown to increase performance and reduce fatigue (23). Resistance training does not deplete as much glycogen as aerobic endurance exercise does (35); however, there is reason to believe that a person dieting for a competition consuming a low-calorie and low-carbohydrate diet and becoming very lean may be glycogen depleted. Therefore, intraworkout consumption of a small amount of fast-digesting carbohydrate (e.g., dextrose) may improve performance. In practice, many people note that they feel this helps gym performance, especially deep in contest prep. Like postworkout protein shake consumption, intraworkout carbohydrate consumption will not negatively affect progress as long as the carbohydrates are accounted for in your daily macronutrient allotment.

One tactic we have used with great results regarding carbohydrate intake flies directly in the face of common bodybuilding lore. Historically, many bodybuilders eliminate nighttime carbohydrates to lose fat. However, we have had success adding a substantial carbohydrate meal before bed for those who have the calories to allow it. A small amount of research shows that this could possibly cause greater fat loss (45). If it does, it is most likely due to improved sleep quality. Since bodybuilders typically have poor sleep quality during contest prep, carbohydrates immediately before bed can be a great tool to improve sleep and therefore improve recovery and fat loss. It should once again be stated that this tactic will only work for those who have enough carbohydrates to spare in their diets, and pretraining carbohydrate intake should always take priority over bedtime carbohydrate consumption.

In summary, we recommend consuming three to six protein-containing meals per day. It would also be advisable to consume one of these meals within one to two hours postworkout (possibly as a postworkout shake) and one before bed. Carbohydrate consumption preworkout should be based on individual tolerance and performance. Moreover, consuming a fast-digesting carbohydrate during a workout may help maintain performance when energy intake and body fat are low. Ultimately, your meal pattern and frequency should allow you to consistently hit your macronutrient numbers each day because without doing so, progress will be suboptimal.

REFEEDS

It is common for competitors to cycle carbohydrate or calorie intake throughout the week. Many believe this helps keep metabolic rate elevated; however, there is limited evidence that a single high-carbohydrate or a high-calorie day has a significant effect on metabolic rate. No published data suggests that complex carbohydrate cycling plans are superior for weight loss versus a consistent carbohydrate intake throughout the week as long as weekly calorie and macronutrient intakes are matched.

But there may be some benefits to incorporating a high-carbohydrate day into your contest prep plan. During periods of low calorie and carbohydrate intake, muscle glycogen stores become depleted. Glycogen in muscle is used for energy during weightlifting, meaning that a depletion of glycogen can reduce performance in the gym. However, a high-carbohydrate day can increase glycogen stores and improve performance during a tough workout (17). Therefore, it may be in your best interest to place a high-carbohydrate refeed day on the day of (or the day before) one of your toughest workout sessions.

Another benefit of a refeed day is that it can allow you to fit in other foods you may be craving. This diet flexibility may reduce the risk of bingeing, thereby improving adherence (44). From an applied standpoint, this mental break is one of the most beneficial effects of a refeed day, even if other claims regarding the benefits of refeeding (such as the effect on metabolic rate) prove to be untrue.

A Structured Refeed Day or a Cheat Day?

Competitors who are dieting for shows often use a refeed day as a "cheat day" or "cheat meal," where they allow themselves to eat anything they want without restriction. However, there are several reasons this is likely not optimal for fat loss and why it would be in your best interest to use a structured refeed day if you are going to include one.

There is no evidence that any individual food causes weight gain or prevents fat loss. Therefore, there is no reason for a healthy competitor to exclude any one food from a diet during contest prep. Instead of eliminating foods or food groups, eat a variety of nutrient-dense foods, fitting in less nutrient-dense foods in moderation while staying within your daily caloric allotment.

And calories from a cheat day still count. Your weight decreases weekly during contest prep if the number of calories consumed throughout the week is lower than the number of calories burned throughout the week. However, if you consume enough calories during your cheat day to offset the calorie deficit created throughout the rest of the week, weight loss will stall.

If a cheat day is turning into an all-out binge, your dietary pattern can begin to look like an eating disorder, where you restrict food for a large portion of the week and a binge on your cheat day. Competing should enhance your life, not detract from it; therefore, you should try to maintain a healthy relationship with food during contest prep.

Uncontrolled cheat days may also make adjustments difficult. As mentioned previously, plateaus are a normal part of weight loss, and they will happen throughout your contest prep. When this occurs, a reduction in caloric intake or increase in activity is necessary to keep weight loss progressing. However, if you incorporate cheat days, the intake on that day may be unclear.

Intake may differ from cheat day to cheat day and increase as you get leaner and hungrier, making meaningful adjustments difficult when plateaus occur.

Many proposed benefits of a high-calorie day during a diet are due to an increased carbohydrate intake. Hormones that affect metabolic rate, such as leptin and thyroid hormone, are much more responsive to carbohydrate overfeeding than to protein or fat overfeeding (5, 38). Therefore, to make the most out of a higher-calorie day, it may be in your best interest to increase carbohydrate intake and not necessarily fat intake as many do during a cheat day.

Refeed Recommendations

For individuals incorporating a refeed day into contest prep, a good starting point would be to increase carbohydrate intake to 1.5 to 2 times your normal intake once every 4 to 10 days. Try to line up refeeds with your hardest workouts so that you are refeeding the day before or the day of your most difficult workout to maximize performance. You may also want to reduce protein and fat intake slightly on your refeed days if caloric intake is low and you notice a large spike in weight after refeeding.

Multiday Refeeds

As mentioned previously, a refeed day does not have a significant lasting effect on metabolic rate or hormones. However, there is some preliminary evidence that having more than one high-calorie or high-carbohydrate day a week may have a greater effect on weight loss (51). Although this topic requires further study, in practice, a few competitors have begun to implement refeeds on two or even three consecutive days with success.

However, weekly caloric intake and energy balance still determine weight change. Therefore, the more refeed days you incorporate, the more caloric intake will need to be reduced on other days.

For example, if you are a female who needs to consume 10,000 calories weekly to see fat loss, your average daily caloric intake for the week needs to be roughly 1,430 calories. If you incorporate a refeed day of 1,700 calories, then your regular days need to be reduced to roughly 1,380 calories to maintain your weekly caloric deficit. However, if you incorporate three consecutive refeeds of 1,700 calories each week, then the remaining four days must be 1,225 calories to maintain your weekly deficit.

As the number of refeeds increase, at some point, you will likely hit a point of diminished returns, where intake on the remaining days is so low that it negatively affects performance in the gym and recovery. This is important to keep in mind if you decide to incorporate multiday refeeds.

DIET BREAKS

Contrary to its name, a diet break is not a free-for-all. Instead, a diet break can be considered a prolonged refeed. Refeeds are a one-, two-, or three-day period where calorie intake is higher, and a diet break is typically one or more weeks of an intake around your current maintenance. This likely has a larger effect on hormone levels and metabolic rate than a refeed day. In addition, it may provide a beneficial mental break from a calorie deficit that can improve motivation and dietary adherence.

The goal of a diet break is not to see weight loss but to hold weight steady. However, preliminary studies have found that a diet break does not affect total weight loss (53) and may even have a beneficial effect on weight loss progress (10).

Therefore, for those with lengthy contest preps, it may not be a bad idea to incorporate diet breaks periodically. This may help keep dietary adherence higher and has beneficial effects on the declines in hormones and metabolic rate that occur during contest prep.

However, we caution about a diet break too close to stage-lean because this essentially prolongs the period in which you stay at an unsustainable body fat and feel the negative effects of contest prep. If you incorporate diet breaks, take them before the final push, when you are feeling the effects of being unsustainably lean.

MONITORING PROGRESS

A variety of strategies can help track of a competitor's progress to lose body fat during the content prep process. Obvious methods are weighing in on a scale and taking progress photos, but monitoring strength levels and measuring body fat can be used also.

Body Weight

To achieve stage-lean levels of body fat, competitors must maintain their target ROLs. Clearly, this means the scale is one method to monitor progress. We recommend weighing in daily to monitor trends and averages over time rather than looking at weight on one specific day.

Weight fluctuations of up to three to five pounds (1.4-2.3 kg) (or even more in some people) from one day to the next are completely normal, even while eating the same thing each day. There are several reasons weight may fluctuate from one day to the next, including sleep patterns, bowel movements, water intake, sweat, stress, hormones, how close you ate to weighing in, and salt intake. However, one thing all these factors have in common is that the changes in weight are the result of water weight or intestinal food mass and not real tissue weight (muscle or fat).

That is why it is important to look at changes in weight over a longer period (i.e., weeks or months) rather than just one day to the next. Look at averages when assessing progress because this can help smooth out some daily fluctuation. We recommend assessing changes in weekly average weights. If your weekly average weight is decreasing at your target ROL, things are likely heading in the right direction.

If you find yourself stressing over the changes from one day to the next, consider weighing in less often. But, weigh yourself more than once a week so that you are not basing adjustments on a single weigh-in each week, which can have a good amount of error. Ultimately, if reducing anxiety about the number on the scale increases your enjoyment of the process, it also will increase the likelihood that you remain consistent and reach your goal.

FAQ: How should a woman handle weight fluctuations due to her menstrual cycle?

Many women have an increase in weight the week before or the week of their monthly menstrual cycles. This fluctuation is due to water weight and is not real tissue weight. If you are a female competitor, note when this fluctuation occurs each month so that you take it into account when assessing your progress. When your weight increases due to your cycle, it will typically be best to continue to stay consistent and see where your weight stabilizes after your cycle. Often, you will be pleased to see that consistency during your cycle has resulted in a nice postcycle loss.

Progress Pictures

Although the scale can be a great marker of progress over the short-term, being stage-lean is not a specific number on the scale; it is a look. Therefore, progress pictures are a key to assessing progress.

However, be honest with your progress pictures. In an age where everything on social media is done with perfect angles, the best lighting, and special filters (and often a good muscle pump too), your progress pictures should not have any of these. You need an honest assessment of how your whole body looks hitting the poses in your division in lighting that may not be "the best." We would also advise not taking progress pictures as a "selfie" using a mirror and instead use consistent lighting and conditions for each set of pictures.

In addition, we would advise against frequent pictures, especially early on in contest prep, because visual progress will take time with slower target ROLs. Therefore, it may be in your best interest to take progress pictures every two to four weeks in the early stages of contest prep, and increase that frequency to every one to two weeks as your competition gets closer.

Strength

Strength loss is common during contest prep, especially in drug-free competitors (39). However, a competitor's goal should be to maintain strength as much as possible during contest prep. Monitoring strength levels can be a great way to assess progress because if the scale is trending down and strength is holding, it is a good sign that you are holding on to muscle mass while dropping body fat. Given enough time and enough change, this should result in the visual changes you are looking for, and your progress pictures will show that as well.

Body Fat Tests

It is common for a competitor with stage-lean levels of body fat to be asked, "What is your body fat percentage?" In reality, this does not matter because the judges are not getting out calipers (or a scale) when you step onstage. We have found that the competitors walking around telling everyone their body fat percentages are not that lean. If they were, they would not need to say anything. It would be obvious.

If you have your body fat measured during contest prep, we advise taking the results with a grain of salt. Studies show that body fat measurements in bodybuilders have quite a bit of error, more than most competitors realize (especially for methods commonly available to competitors, such as bioelectrical impedance analysis) (50). This means that the number the test gives you may be significantly different than your true body fat. It also means that you are going to need to see a large change in body fat between measurements to be sure that the difference in body fat measured is real body fat loss and not just a random measurement error. To minimize error in body fat measurements as much as possible, use more precise measurement techniques, such as dual-energy X-ray absorptiometry (DEXA).

Regardless of the technique that you use, take your measurement at the same time and under the same conditions. Typically, it is easiest to do this first thing in the morning before eating, wearing minimal clothing, and after emptying your bladder. It is also best that you do not have a refeed day the day before your measurement to minimize water and glycogen fluctuation.

Although a test's standardization reduces the error of the measurement, all measurements have error. If you take body composition measurements during contest prep, do not label your prep as a success or a failure based on body fat measurement numbers. Take the results in context with body weight, visual results, and strength changes to get a full picture of what is happening during your contest prep.

PLATEAUS

Plateaus are a normal part of the fat-loss process. During contest prep, you can expect to hit several plateaus. These plateaus occur due to the body's metabolic adaptation from several factors, such as weight loss, lean mass loss, reduced voluntary and involuntary movement outside the gym (also known as NEAT, nonexercise adaptive thermogenesis), reduced hormone levels (e.g., leptin, thyroid, testosterone, and estrogen), increased mitochondrial efficiency, and increased extraction of nutrients by the microbes in the GI tract (as reviewed by 30, 49).

Making Adjustments

If you are not losing weight, you need to reduce intake, increase activity, or both to create an energy deficit again. Double-check that you are consistently following the plan. This includes consistently meeting your macronutrient numbers and getting in all cardio and workouts. Perhaps the biggest thing to double-check is whether you are tracking your nutritional intake accurately and not underreporting calories, something very common (28, 29) even in trained dietitians (13). For this reason, ensuring you are accurately accounting for everything you are eating is incredibly important. If you find that you have not been consistent, keep everything as is and focus on consistency first before determining if adjustments are necessary.

If you are accounting for everything you are consuming, being consistent with your macro numbers, and getting all your workouts in and still not losing weight, then you need to decrease your caloric intake, increase your activity level, or both to get you back into an energy deficit. We discuss adjustments to both exercise and nonexercise activity in the next chapter. However, for now, we will focus on changes in energy intake.

It is a common mistake to make large adjustments each time a plateau occurs. However, often only a small adjustment (50-150 calories per day) is necessary to keep weight loss moving appropriately. Reduce these calories from carbohydrate (and possibly fat) while keeping protein high to protect against muscle loss.

Ultimately, your goal should be to keep caloric intake as high as possible while still seeing an appropriate ROL. This way, there is room to make further adjustments if or when additional plateaus occur along the way. Always having something in your back pocket that you can pull out when a plateau occurs will ensure that you can continue to lose weight and progress toward your goal of looking your best onstage.

Take-Home Points

► Aim for 0.5 to 1 percent of body weight loss weekly on average, sticking to the lower end of this range if possible. Consume as many calories as possible while seeing this ROL.

► Consume 1 to 1.4 grams of protein per pound of lean body weight, 20 to 30 percent of calories from fat, and the remainder of your daily caloric allotment from carbohydrate while eating at least 10 to 14 grams of fiber per 1,000 calories consumed. Be aware that this is a good starting point for many, but not necessarily a one-size-fits-all, and some competitors may need a different macronutrient breakdown for optimal progress.

► There is no need to eliminate any food, food group, or macronutrient unless you have a diagnosed medical reason to do so. Instead, eat a variety of foods from all food groups to prevent vitamin and mineral deficiencies.

► Consume three to six protein-containing meals daily with special attention to protein post-workout and before bed. Base preworkout and intraworkout carbohydrate intake on tolerance and performance in the gym.

► Consider incorporating a higher-carbohydrate day every 4 to 10 days to help performance during a tough workout and provide a mental break. There may also be added benefits to multiple high-carbohydrate days in a row or a diet break periodically during contest prep.

► Plateaus are a normal part of the weight loss process. When they occur, reduce caloric intake only a small amount (primarily from carbohydrate and fat in most cases) to restore target rate of weekly loss while consuming as many calories as possible.

Tweaking Your Physique for Contest Preparation

7

As mentioned earlier, to maintain your target ROL during contest prep, you need to be in an energy deficit, where energy intake is lower than energy expenditure. In the previous chapter, we discussed how to adjust your nutrition plan to reduce energy intake while holding on to as much muscle mass as possible during contest prep. In this chapter, we discuss the components of energy expenditure: exercise and nonexercise activity. We also focus on how to create an effective resistance training plan to minimize muscle loss during contest prep.

INCREASING ENERGY EXPENDITURE

It is important to consider energy expenditure, not just calorie reduction, when attempting to create an energy deficit. A plan to burn calories inside and outside the gym will support your bodybuilding efforts, giving you the lean look you seek. The two most modifiable components of total daily energy expenditure are exercise and nonexercise activity.

Cardio Training

The most common way to increase exercise energy expenditure is by adding cardio. Historically, bodybuilders add a lot of cardio when starting contest prep to create a significant energy deficit and achieve a rapid ROL. However, you should shoot for slower ROLs than bodybuilders have historically; therefore, these extremes likely are not necessary for most competitors. This section outlines an evidence-based approach to adding cardio during contest prep.

Amount of Cardio

It is entirely possible to create an energy deficit without cardio; however, this is not realistic for most people because it would require an extremely low caloric intake that may make dietary adherence difficult. In addition, an extremely low intake may adversely affect performance in the gym and recovery between workouts. Therefore, for most competitors, some level of cardio is necessary.

Historically, bodybuilders have done long durations of cardio daily from the start of contest prep. However, this may not be optimal for muscle retention while dieting. In fact, a study found that the more cardio a person does, the more it interferes with strength and size gains from lifting

71

weights (44). This interference may be greater in advanced athletes (most people stepping onstage would be considered advanced athletes if they are giving themselves adequate training time before a show) (5).

Taken together, this suggests that you should aim to do as little cardio as possible while still seeing your target rate of weight loss. This does not mean you will be doing no cardio, and most competitors require cardio to get stage-lean. However, it will be in your best interest to achieve your target ROL on as little cardio as necessary at a given time. If you can get stage-lean through caloric changes only, then we would recommend that you do so, but if you are not so lucky, then you should keep cardio as low as possible during prep.

FAQ: Should I do cardio fasted?

Doing cardio first thing in the morning before eating is commonly the cardio choice of bodybuilders because they believe that it results in greater fat loss. However, a study directly comparing fasted- and fed-state cardio observed no difference in weight loss, fat loss, or body composition (28). Therefore, competitors can feel free to perform cardio fasted or fed based on individual preference.

Intensity of Cardio

Many individuals do lower-intensity forms of cardio because more fat is burned during exercise; however, studies comparing low- and high-intensity forms of cardio observed no difference in fat burned throughout the day (20, 27). This is because a greater amount of fat is burned following higher-intensity forms of cardio. In addition, high-intensity cardio interferes less with strength and size gains (44).

Before switching to an exclusively high-intensity cardio plan, there are other considerations. High-intensity cardio is more difficult to recover from than lower-intensity forms. Recovery ability may be reduced in a caloric deficit, where recovery abilities are not as high as in the off-season. In addition, the high intensity may cause issues with preexisting joint conditions or even create joint or injury issues if the amount of high-intensity cardio performed exceeds recovery ability.

Another consideration is that research on high-intensity cardio and interference with strength and size gains was not conducted on dieting bodybuilders who have fuel in short supply. From a practical standpoint, high-intensity cardio can be problematic for a bodybuilder in prep. The primary fuel source for intense resistance training is glucose. Glucose is also the primary fuel for high-intensity cardio. Therefore, performing high-intensity cardio robs fuel from your resistance training. In the off-season, when a bodybuilder is adequately fed, this is not a problem. However, during a contest prep, when calories and carbohydrates are restricted, this can be a big problem. Also, recovery ability is already hindered during contest prep, and high-intensity cardio can worsen the situation. On the other hand, little recovery is needed after going for a 30-minute walk.

Because high-intensity cardio can take away fuel from your resistance training and then hinder recovery from resistance training, we recommend that you use high-intensity cardio very sparingly or possibly reduce or eliminate its use entirely as a contest prep progresses and calories get lower. It is not uncommon to only tolerate one or two high-intensity interval training sessions weekly without affecting performance. From there, you should add steady-state cardio for any additional cardio needs. Many people may not do well with high-intensity cardio and may need to stick to low- and moderate-cardio intensities instead.

FAQ: If I am lifting weights and doing cardio in the same workout, which should I do first?

At times during contest prep, it may be necessary to perform cardio and resistance training in the same session. In this circumstance, it will be in your best interest to perform weights before cardio. Performing cardio immediately before resistance training has been shown to reduce strength gain (25). Performing cardio after resistance training lowers injury risk versus performing resistance training following an intense cardio session. For example, think about trying to perform heavy barbell squats after a high-intensity interval session of sprints.

It is important to space out higher-intensity forms of cardio and resistance training workouts using the same muscle groups. For example, we would recommend not doing a high-intensity interval cardio session on the spin bike the day before performing heavy squats.

Nonexercise Activity Thermogenesis

Most competitors only think "cardio" when discussing ways to increase energy expenditure. However, nonexercise activity can play a huge role in creating an energy deficit and maintaining target ROL. NEAT is all other movement you do outside the gym. This includes voluntary activity, like work, cleaning, shopping, recreational activity, or walking a pet as well as involuntary activity like twitching and fidgeting.

There are large person-to-person variations in NEAT (17). Much of the variation is due to differences in profession. Clearly, it is not realistic to change your profession just to diet for a bodybuilding competition, and you cannot change how much you fidget; however, you can make a conscious effort to move more throughout the day outside of your time in the gym.

Role of NEAT in Bodybuilding

During contest prep, when you are extremely lean and energy intake is low, NEAT will decrease to conserve energy (13). This reduction is a large contributor to metabolic adaptation and the weight loss plateaus normal to the dieting process (18, 40). For those who have been stage-lean, this likely makes complete sense. You can relate to the fact that you move less when stage-lean because you feel tired and sluggish. However, this only reduces your total daily energy expenditure. Therefore, stay active outside the gym and keep NEAT elevated during contest prep.

Increasing NEAT During Contest Prep

One effective way to increase NEAT is to track daily steps (3). This can be done using fancy watches, cell phone apps, or even a cheap, old-school pedometer. Regardless of the tracking method, you need to first get an idea of your baseline daily activity levels. If you work an active job, you likely average over 10,000 steps daily. Those with sedentary jobs often fall in the 5,000- to 7,000-step range, and individuals who work sedentary jobs from home can average as low as 2,000 to 4,000 steps daily.

Once you have an idea of your average daily step count, you need to set a daily step minimum. It is a good idea to set a step minimum slightly above your current activity but not extremely higher. This makes your starting daily step minimum doable, increases energy expenditure a bit, and gives you room to increase NEAT throughout prep as necessary. For example, if you are averaging 6,700 steps daily, a good starting step minimum may be around 8,000 steps per day.

You need to find ways to increase your daily activity to hit these numbers. This could be from things like going for a walk, going to the store, walking a pet, playing with your kids, cleaning your house, parking further away, taking the stairs, or any other type of activity throughout the day. However, the goal will be to get your steps in with lower-intensity activity to keep NEAT high and not impact your performance in the gym.

Benefits of NEAT

There are a few benefits to tracking NEAT during contest prep. One is that it is a way to increase energy expenditure to help you maintain ROL. It can also be done anywhere throughout the day and does not require more time in the gym. For busy people, this is a huge bonus.

NEAT is also lower-intensity than formal cardio and should not interfere as much with performance and recovery in the gym. For example, you likely cannot do more than one or two high-intensity interval training sessions a week and still recover for your workouts; however, you can walk a few thousand extra steps each day with little to no effect on performance in the gym.

Finally, by tracking steps and increasing activity, you can help offset some reduction in NEAT that occurs during prep. This does not completely prevent plateaus, and they will still be a normal part of the dieting process. However, you limit a major factor leading to weight loss plateaus.

Adjustments to Create an Energy Deficit

As discussed previously, plateaus occur for several reasons (40). When they occur, you need to adjust to create an energy deficit and continue to reach your target ROL. One way to create an energy deficit is to reduce calorie intake as outlined in the previous chapter. However, energy expenditure can also be altered through addition of cardio and NEAT.

In general, your goal during contest prep should be to get away with as much food and as little cardio or other activity as possible while still seeing progress. For this reason, we would recommend only adding small amounts of cardio at a time when adjusting. You may also want to hold off on adding extra cardio until intake is lower to keep performance and recovery in the gym as high as possible.

In addition, it may be in your best interest to adjust step counts first before adding in formal cardio sessions because lower-intensity activity (e.g., walking) is easier to recover from than added cardio. Often, adding 1,000 to 2,000 steps to your daily step minimum can be a powerful tool along with a reduction in intake to create an energy deficit and increase ROL.

However, we would caution adding extreme amounts of steps or cardio just to be able to eat more food. Although this may result in an energy deficit and weight loss, it may interfere with performance and recovery in the gym. In addition, there is evidence that you get less added value from added activity when activity levels are already extremely high (24). It is thought that this is due to a reduction in the involuntary components of NEAT to conserve energy. It also means that the extra 30 to 60 minutes of weekly cardio time or 1,000 to 2,000 additional steps may not have as much benefit when activity levels are extremely high as they would when activity is at a more reasonable level.

In the end, cardio and daily step counts are tools that can be used to create an energy deficit. However, like any tool, they need to be used appropriately for the best results. Add cardio and steps as necessary, but do not abuse these tools to eat significantly more food. You may end up impairing your recovery and losing strength and, ultimately, muscle mass during contest prep.

RESISTANCE TRAINING

Although resistance training does not expend as many calories as cardio, lifting weights should be the focus of a competitor's time in the gym. It provides a stimulus for muscle maintenance during contest prep. One common mistake competitors make is backing off their efforts in the gym during contest prep; however, this is a recipe for muscle loss. Therefore, it is important to understand the variables to consider when programming training and how to construct an effective resistance training program during contest prep.

Program Design Variables

Each factor in a resistance training program has a specific effect on the body and the results you get from your program. The overarching goal is to force your body to handle more work over time, a strategy called **progressive overload**. Adding more work continues to provide a new and greater stimulus that the body must then adapt to. Progressive overload should remain the primary focus of a resistance training program during contest prep. Progression can be achieved in several ways, such as increasing weight used, reps performed, volume lifted, or proximity to failure, or even by performing the same weight, sets, and reps on a movement with better technique. However, the key is that you are aiming for progression over time in some aspect of your workouts.

For most people, gaining strength while stage-lean is not possible. In fact, most competitors (especially those who are drug-free) lose strength during contest prep (26). However, the goal in the gym should be to lift as heavy as possible while maintaining proper technique and aiming to progress where you are able.

The following sections describe each program design variable that, when combined, result in a well-rounded and effective resistance training program.

Exercise Selection

The first consideration when constructing a training plan is to determine which exercises you are going to do. This is likely going to differ from person to person. However, you have a physique-based goal, so there is no exercise that you *must* do as long as you are training each muscle group. The barbell back squat, barbell deadlift, and barbell bench press are great movements; if you have an injury that keeps you from being able to do any of these movements pain-free, though, you do not have to incorporate them to make progress. However, it would be in your best interest to verify that your pain or injury is not caused by a technique flaw before excluding the exercise completely.

Assuming that form is not the issue, you can always find a similar alternative for movements that cause pain. Does your back hurt when you do a barbell back squat? That is OK because you may do things like single-leg dumbbell-loaded squatting and lunging movements, leg press, hack squat, leg extensions, hip thrust, hamstring curls, and many other lower body movements without pain. You may even be able to still squat with lighter weight and higher reps. But if an exercise causes pain, do not do it.

In addition, you should perform exercises for which you are able to use good form throughout a full range of motion. This increases muscle recruitment and strength and, ultimately, reduces injury risk (19, 38). Ensure that you can do a movement through a full range of motion with good technique before doing heavy loads.

You also want to incorporate a variety of movements to target a given muscle group from different angles. In fact, a study found that a workout that incorporated squats, leg presses, and lunges resulted in more balanced muscle growth than the same number of working sets from squats alone (8). For complete development, focus on several different movements per muscle group.

One final factor in your exercise selection is the principle of **specificity**. This means that you must train specific to your goals. If your goal is to improve development in certain muscle groups, then your exercises should target those areas to the greatest degree. For example, while a barbell bent-over row taxes the rear delts, it is not the primary muscle group being trained in that exercise. If you wish to specifically focus on the rear delts, you need to perform exercises where that muscle group is the primary area of focus, such as a bent-over lateral raise or a reverse pec dec fly. When choosing your exercises, make sure to always keep your goals in mind, and then train specific to those goals.

FAQ: What is the mind-muscle connection I have heard about?

Referring to the mind-muscle connection in bodybuilding can quickly sound like you are advocating some sort of voodoo magic if you are not careful. However, this is an old-school idea finally getting some new-school science behind it. The idea behind the mind-muscle connection is that you should be able to "feel" the muscle working when you train it. It is not enough to mindlessly move a weight from point A to point B and back again. You should focus on feeling the target muscle working and flexing it as you work it. This is called training with intent.

While the mind-muscle connection has largely just been an anecdotal observation throughout the decades, there is some new research showing that lifting with intent indeed increases muscular growth (35). It turns out the old-school bodybuilders had this one right all along! Properly tapping into the mind-muscle connection can come down to several variables. Exercise selection is indeed important. You should do movements that you feel instead of movements that do not provide that sensation or cause that awareness. You should always aim to improve your technique to feel the target muscle group to a greater degree. Another factor is to flex the muscle against the weight as you lift and to think about that muscle as you train it. Overall, a good rule of thumb is that if you do not feel a muscle when you are training it, you likely are not activating it optimally.

Frequency

Once you have an idea of the exercises you will perform in the gym, the next variable to consider is how frequently you are going to do them or train a specific muscle group. It is common in the bodybuilding world to train each muscle group once a week; however, this is not the only way to structure workouts.

The scientific literature shows muscle protein synthesis rates are elevated 36 to 48 hours (at most) following a workout in trained individuals (23). This means that the rate at which your body is repairing and growing muscle tissue increases for a 36- to 48-hour period after you train each muscle group. Based on these results, it may be beneficial to train muscle groups more than once a week to keep protein synthesis rates elevated for a greater period. Indeed, studies have found that training each muscle group at least twice weekly is superior for muscle growth, even when weekly training volume is matched (31).

However, before you use these results to justify training your whole body every day, there are some other considerations. Researchers in this study were not able to identify additional benefit of training muscle groups more than two times weekly. There is evidence that tendon turnover is a longer process than muscle tissue turnover. Whereas protein synthesis levels in muscles return to baseline in 36 to 48 hours, elevated tendon protein synthesis levels have been observed 72 hours after exercise (21). This means tendons take longer to recover from resistance training than muscle tissue does. Therefore, extremely high training frequencies may increase risk of overuse injury. As a result, training frequencies of two or three times weekly are recommended for trained individuals (41).

When increasing training frequency, keep weekly training volume the same. For example, if you normally do 10 sets of chest exercises once weekly, begin by doing 5 sets of chest exercises twice weekly rather than doing 10 sets of chest exercises twice weekly. Doubling weekly training volume is likely unnecessary and increases injury risk. Therefore, it will be in your best interest to increase training frequency while keeping the amount of work you are doing for the week constant.

FAQ: How many days a week should I be in the gym?

There is no magical number of days per week you need to be in the gym. Base the number of workouts you are doing weekly on what is necessary to achieve your desired training volume and cardio. Also, make sure that you are basing your weekly schedule on your recovery ability in the gym and personal schedule outside the gym. Contest prep should not be an excuse to ignore everything else going on in your real life.

Volume

Volume is the number of sets or the product of the number of sets, reps, and weight someone performs or lifts for a given exercise or workout. In the bodybuilding world, there are a number of theories in terms of the most optimal volume for muscle growth, ranging from workouts with one working set per muscle group to those where people may be in the gym for three or four hours to absolutely crush themselves.

An analysis of studies examining training volume and muscle growth concluded that multiple-set workouts are superior to single-set workouts for muscle growth (15). This means the old-school high-intensity training protocol of one set to failure is not optimal for muscle growth. In addition, an analysis found that doing 10 or more sets weekly per muscle group was superior for muscle growth to doing fewer than 10 working sets weekly (30).

Although this makes a strong case that doing more is always better, more volume is only better to a point. As you continue to add volume, you will see less benefit from the added training volume. If you push training volume far enough, you may not achieve any additional benefit for the extra volume. Moreover, if volume is taken even further to the point you are not able to recover, you may observe less progress or, even worse, get injured as a result. Therefore, more is only better as long as you are still able to recover.

There is also some evidence of this in the scientific literature (1). A study comparing 5 and 10 sets per exercise found that over the course of six weeks, participants in the 5-set group made greater increases in many measures of muscle size and strength. This is likely due to the 10 sets per exercise protocol pushing participants beyond their recovery capacities.

You should adjust training volume based on your individual recovery ability, keeping in mind that recovery may be reduced deep in prep when intake is lower, cardio is higher, and body fat is low. Pay attention to how you are feeling, recovering, and progressing in the gym when assessing your training volume.

Exercise Order

Once you have a list of movements you want to do on a given day and know how much volume you are aiming for, you need to determine the order that you perform those exercises. You can perform more volume with exercises earlier in the workout (37). Therefore, along with increasing frequency and volume for weaknesses, you may want to arrange exercises within a workout to target weaknesses first when you are fresh and can achieve the most volume.

Repetition Range

It is typically thought that the 1 to 5 repetition range is the best for strength, 6 to 12 or 8 to 15 is best for hypertrophy, and more than 15 is best for endurance. As a result, many bodybuilders train exclusively in the 6 to 12 or 8 to 15 repetition range.

However, muscle growth can be achieved across a wide array of repetition ranges. In fact, several studies have observed that when **volume load** (sets × reps × weight) is matched, repetition ranges of 6 or fewer reps result in similar hypertrophy to sets of 8 to 12 (4, 14, 34). Moreover, sets taken to failure in the 25- to 35-rep range result in similar hypertrophy to the 8- to 12-rep range

(22, 32). Additionally, more growth may be achieved when training with a variety of repetition ranges (8, 29).

Therefore, it will be in your best interest to focus on progression over a variety of repetition ranges for optimal muscle growth. This can be done in several ways, such as training muscle groups in a lower-repetition range early in the week and a higher-repetition range later in the week or training movements earlier in your workout in lower-repetition ranges with movements later in the workout in higher-repetition ranges.

Rest Period Length

It is common to see hypertrophy-based workouts include short rest periods of 30 to 60 seconds, likely because shorter rest periods between sets result in a greater acute increase in hormones such as growth hormone. However, there is no evidence that acute physiological changes in hormones occurring during a workout correlate with muscle growth (42). Planning workouts to maximize acute hormone change will not influence muscle growth.

Additionally, a review on rest periods and muscle hypertrophy concluded that rest periods have no effect on muscle hypertrophy if training volume is matched (11). A study observed less growth with one-minute rest periods compared with three-minute rest periods (33). This likely occurred because greater training volume can be achieved with longer rest periods. For example, someone performing three sets of 10 reps on barbell back squat resting as necessary may only be able to achieve 10, 7, and 5 reps on the three sets, respectively, if rest was reduced to one minute. A total of 22 reps in the short rest condition compared to 30 reps in the longer rest condition means the longer rest condition would result in more training volume and growth.

Although there may be a time and place for shorter rest periods in a training program, in general, it is best to take the amount of time you need between sets to recover and have a quality performance on your next set. This keeps you injury-free and progressing.

FAQ: Do I need to train to failure? If so, should I do it in every workout?

It is common for physique athletes to train to failure. While training to failure increases muscle recruitment, it also increases injury risk, is more difficult to recover from, and is not required for muscle growth (43). An analysis examining the relationship between training to failure and muscle growth found no difference between the failure and subfailure conditions. In fact, the existing literature suggests that there may be slightly more growth in the subfailure condition as opposed to training to failure (6).

This does not mean that training to failure is useless. It is a tool, and like any tool, it may be useful in the appropriate situation. When training to failure, be smart about picking when and how often this tool is implemented. It may be best to incorporate training to absolute failure primarily on isolation exercises (e.g., leg extension) rather than on full-body compound movements (e.g., squat) to prevent injury risk and help recovery.

Repetition Tempo

Very slow training was popular in the 1980s and 1990s. Today, some bodybuilders still do it. However, aside from uses in tendon rehabilitation (16), the data on extremely slow eccentric training for bodybuilders is not strong. Super slow training has been shown to result in less muscle activation (7), metabolic stress (7), training volume (10), strength gain (12), and muscle growth (36) than a traditional repetition tempo of approximately one to three seconds for the eccentric part of the movement.

Much like training to failure, slow eccentrics are a tool that may be beneficial in certain situations; however, it is not ideal to *always* use extremely slow repetition tempos. This does not mean your form should be sloppy. In fact, there is evidence that proper form can increase muscle activation (38). Poor form and sloppy reps increase your injury risk. When you are lifting weights, you should control the weights throughout the entire range of motion, but there is no need to do very slow reps on everything.

Workout Length

Many people cap workouts at a certain point due to a fear of "going catabolic." However, there is no evidence this occurs. In fact, a study looking at the correlation between changes in hormones during a workout and muscle growth observed a slight positive correlation between cortisol increase and muscle growth (42). This likely occurred because hard training acutely increases muscle growth and cortisol—not necessarily because increased cortisol was causing muscle growth. However, the take-home point from this study is that you can take as long as you need to get your training volume in. There is no need to cap workout length, but it is important to keep training volumes within your recovery ability.

Program Design Summary

A good starting point when designing a training program is to target each muscle group with at least 10 sets weekly. Ensure your volume is an amount that you can recover from and emphasize more volume toward weaker muscle groups and less toward strengths. Organize your volume per muscle group into two or three sessions weekly. Train with a variety of repetition ranges, implementing tools such as failure, short rest periods, slower reps, and other intensity techniques in an organized manner if you decide to include them in your plan.

Other Considerations

The previous recommendations provide a general evidence-based framework for constructing a resistance training plan; however, you need to consider several other practical variables to make the most out of your training program.

Enjoyment

This is an often-overlooked factor when designing a training program. If you are trying to do what is in theory the "best" program for you but do not enjoy it, the odds are you are not going to work as hard or stay as consistent. Therefore, you may not reach your goals. However, if you implement some things you enjoy doing (within reason), along with what should help to make the most progress, you may enjoy the program more and work harder.

Flexibility

Bodybuilders can vary greatly in the amount of structure they prefer in their workouts. Do you like to have every detail (sets, reps, weight, rest period, tempo, etc.) programmed out for you, or does the thought of that make you absolutely dread heading to the gym?

Those who enjoy every detail programmed out should do that. Those who prefer having a bit more flexibility may find a good middle ground if they have a programmed progression for their main exercises with a few exercise options or a volume total for their assistance work.

Ultimately, if you look at your plan and dread going into the gym to do it, you are not going to work as hard. Give yourself the flexibility you need in your program to stay sane yet be sure to still have enough structure so that you progress over time.

Life Stressors

At times, people attempt workouts far beyond what their schedules or recovery abilities allow. This can lead to reduced consistency, fewer gains, and, worst case, an injury.

Is your job a physical one? If so, you may want to consider training with less volume so that you are able to recover.

Are you under a lot of stress and not getting enough sleep? If so, you may want to consider training with less volume because high stress levels can impair recovery from workouts and reduce progress over time (2, 39).

Are you only able to realistically be in the gym three days per week? You can still make great progress if you do not set up a five-day split for yourself.

As you are setting up your plan, be sure you also consider your real-life schedule and other stressors in your life so you recover and progress toward your goals.

MONITOR THE NEED FOR RECOVERY

As discussed, during contest prep, when a competitor is in a caloric deficit, his or her recovery ability is not as high as what it is in the off-season, especially if cardio is higher and body fat is low. Therefore, be aware of symptoms that indicate an overreached state and make necessary adjustments to the training program, such as deloading.

Address Overreaching

Bodybuilders train hard; however, at some point, you will exceed your recovery ability as fatigue from training begins to accumulate. You may notice that you do not have quite as much motivation in the gym, little injuries start to pop up, you do not sleep as well, strength is not increasing like it had been, or you simply do not feel recovered in the gym. This is **overreaching** and may have a benefit in the context of a properly designed program.

Respond to overreaching when it occurs rather than pushing through to the point where you have a major injury or become overtrained. Recovering from an overtrained state takes far longer than recovering from overreaching, so monitor your performance in the gym and need for recovery to address overreaching when it occurs (9).

Deload

The easiest way to address overreaching is to perform a deload week. During this time, training volume or intensity (or both) is reduced. If you feel run-down, it may not be a bad idea to take a few extra days off from the gym during your deload week as well; you will tend to recover faster when skipping the gym completely rather than doing light workouts.

However, do not lower your caloric intake during this week, even though training volume is lower. Lowering energy intake during a deload week may negatively affect your ability to recover.

Back off in the gym when necessary rather than trying to push through. Contest prep will be difficult—there is no reason to make it more difficult than it needs to be and sacrifice results to be more hard-core than your competition.

SAMPLE TRAINING PROGRAMS

In this chapter, we discussed many variables to consider when designing a training program. There are an infinite number of ways to organize these variables into an effective training plan. We have included three examples of ways to organize your training. However, much like with the sample meals plans in the previous chapter, the best program for you will depend on the factors covered earlier in this chapter.

Power Block Periodization Program

Power block periodization is a hybrid between traditional powerlifting-style workouts with heavy weights on squat, bench, and deadlift (powerlifting days) and traditional bodybuilding-style workouts with higher reps (block training days). It is a five-day-a-week program with a full-body lower-repetition power day to begin the week and four workouts later in the week with a higher split by muscle group (table 7.1).

Specific exercises to perform each day can be found in table 7.2. In this example, there is a relatively even focus among all muscle groups; however, this workout could easily be modified based on your weaknesses and can easily be adjusted in the assistance exercises performed on the powerlifting day. Another option is to perform extra sets for weaknesses and fewer sets for strengths on block training days.

Powerlifting Days

When starting this plan, know your 1 repetition max (1RM) or at least an estimated 1RM for your squat, bench press, and deadlift. Once you determine these numbers, subtract 20 to 25 pounds (9-11 kg) from your 1RM and use that as your starting max for the program. This allows you to build momentum for several weeks. For example, if you can squat 300 pounds (136 kg), then your 1RM to start this plan will be 275 pounds (125 kg).

Table 7.1   Sample Power Block Periodization Weekly Training Split

WEEK	DAY 1	DAY 2	DAY 3	DAY 4	DAY 5	DAY 6	DAY 7
1	Powerlifting day	Off	Legs, shoulders	Back, traps, biceps	Chest, triceps, abs	Legs, shoulders	Off
2	Powerlifting day	Off	Back, traps, biceps	Chest, triceps, abs	Legs, shoulders	Back, traps, biceps	Off
3	Powerlifting day	Off	Chest, triceps, abs	Legs, shoulders	Back, traps, biceps	Chest, triceps, abs	Off

Table 7.2   Sample Power Block Periodization Program

POWERLIFTING DAY	BLOCK TRAINING DAYS		
Squat: 2 × 5 @ 70% 2 × 3 @ 80% 1 × 1 @ 90% **Bench:** 2 × 5 @ 70% 2 × 3 @ 80% 1 × 1 @ 90% **Deadlift:** 2 × 5 @ 70% 2 × 3 @ 80% 1 × 1 @ 90% **As many as possible @ 90%:** DB bench press: 2-3 × 4-6 Cable row: 2-3 × 4-6 Hamstring curl: 2-3 × 4-6 Calf raise: 2-3 × 4-6	**Legs, shoulders**	**Back, traps, biceps**	**Chest, triceps, abs**
	Hack squat: 4 sets	T-bar row: 4 sets	Incline DB bench press: 3 sets
	Leg press: 2 sets	Pull-up: 5 sets	Machine bench press: 4 sets
	Leg extension: 4 sets	Cable row: 4 sets	Cable fly: 4 sets
	Hamstring curl: 3 sets	Deadlift: 2 sets	Cable pressdown: 4 sets
	Walking lunge: 2 sets	DB shrug: 3 sets	Overhead triceps extension: 4 sets
	Calf raise: 4 sets	DB curl: 4 sets	Abs: 3 sets
	DB overhead press: 3 sets	Preacher curl: 2 sets	
	Side lateral raise: 3 sets	Hammer curl: 2 sets	
	DB rear lateral raise: 3 sets		

On your last set of squat, bench, and deadlift, attempt to complete as many reps as possible while not hitting failure. If you can complete 3 reps or more on your last set, the following week, add five pounds (2 kg) to your 1RM and recalculate your numbers. If you fail to complete 3 reps on your last set, use the same numbers for the following week. If you fail to accomplish 3 reps on your last set for two consecutive weeks, lower your 1RM by 20 pounds (9 kg) and recalculate the following week. This is a continuous cycle.

Block Training Days

For the block training days, adjust the repetition ranges every three weeks as follows:

- ► Weeks 1-3: 5-7 reps
- ► Weeks 4-6: 8-10 reps
- ► Weeks 7-9: 10-15 reps
- ► Weeks 10-12: 15-30 reps

We also recommend deloading on week 13 after completing 12 weeks of this program. Also, if you feel run-down at any point in this program, be sure you are taking a deload week early.

Blood Volume Maximum Overload Program

This plan is more like what most would think of when they think of a "bodybuilding" training program. It incorporates higher reps and pump work but also has some heavier loads included. Six workouts (table 7.3) will be rotated in a three on, one off, two on, one off pattern so you do not train the same muscle group on the same day each week.

Blood Volume Workouts

The goal of blood volume training is to force as much blood into the muscle as possible. This is done by high reps, supersets, and constant tension on the muscle. During blood volume workouts, perform the reps slowly. It should take you a full three seconds to lift the weight and a full three seconds to lower the weight. At the contracted position, you should squeeze the muscle very hard. Rest no longer than 10 seconds between exercises within a superset and 1 to 1.5 minutes between supersets. If you cannot perform the prescribed number of reps, lower the weight. This type of training should be extremely painful. If it is not, increase the weight or slow down the repetition.

Overload Workouts

The primary goal of overload workouts is to get stronger and break personal records. Every working set should be taken to within one or two reps of failure. For the first two weeks of this program, do not go to failure. On week three, take one set for each body part to failure, and on week four, take the last set of every exercise to failure. When choosing your weight, pick one with which you can perform at least four reps but no more than seven reps. Once you can perform seven reps with a given weight, increase the weight on the following workout. Rest periods should be two to four minutes in length.

Bikini Division Training Program

The prior sample workouts focused evenly on all muscle groups. However, as mentioned, some divisions place greater emphasis on certain muscle groups. For example, the bikini division places a large emphasis on the lower body, glutes, back, and shoulders. The sample program provided in tables 7.4 to 7.6 is one example of how to organize training that focuses on those specific muscle groups. A similar approach of emphasizing weaknesses and deemphasizing strengths can be used for competitors who are working to strengthen weak muscle groups.

The sample bikini training program alternates between low-repetition (4-8), moderate-repetition (6-15), and high-repetition (15-30) workouts. It is also organized in three, three-week waves. Volume increases over the course of each three-week wave, and the repetition ranges decrease every three weeks (with a corresponding increase in the loads lifted). After completing the nine weeks of training, we recommend deloading in week 10.

Table 7.3   Sample Blood Volume Maximum Overload Training Program

Workout 1	
Back and traps (Overload)	Deadlift 3 × 4-7
	Pull-up 3 × 4-7
	Lat pulldown 3 × 4-7
	T-Bar row 3 × 4-7
	Low machine row 3 × 4-7
	Barbell shrug 2 × 4-7
Delts (blood volume)	DB lateral raise 4 × 14-20 superset with DB overhead press 4 × 14-20
	Rear delt machine fly 3 × 14-20 superset with upright row 3 × 14-20
Workout 2	
Legs (blood volume)	Leg extension 4 × 14-20 superset with leg press 4 × 14-20
	Hamstring curl 4 × 14-20 superset with hack squat 4 × 14-20
	Barbell hip thrust 2 × 14-20
	DB calf raise 2 × 14-20 superset with toe press 2 × 14-20
Abdominals (blood volume)	Sit-up 3 × 14-20
	Cable crunch 3 × 14-20
Workout 3	
Chest (overload)	Bench press 3 × 4-7
	Decline bench 3 × 4-7
	DB incline press 3 × 4-7
	Pec dec machine 3 × 4-7
Biceps (blood volume)	Hammer curl 3 × 14-20 superset with barbell curl 3 × 14-20
	Wide DB curl 3 × 14-20 superset with cable curl 3 × 14-20
Triceps (blood volume)	V-bar cable pushdown 3 × 14-20 superset with DB skullcrusher 3 × 14-20
	2-arm DB kickback 3 × 14-20 superset with machine triceps extension 3 × 14-20
Workout 4	
Delts (overload)	DB military press 3 × 4-7
	DB lateral raise 3 × 4-7
	Reverse pec dec 3 × 4-7
	Barbell upright row 3 × 4-7
Back and traps (blood volume)	Neutral grip cable row 4 × 14-20 superset with standing DB row 4 × 14-20
	Machine row 4 × 14-20 superset with neutral grip lat pulldown 4 × 14-20
	DB shrug 1 × 14-20 superset with straight-bar cable shrug 1 × 14-20
Workout 5	
Legs (overload)	Squat 3 × 4-7
	Leg extension 3 × 4-7

(continued)

Table 7.3 *(continued)*

Workout 5		
	DB leg curl 3 × 4-7	
	Stiff-leg deadlift 3 × 4-7	
	DB walking lunge 1 × 7-10 (each leg)	
	Hip abduction 2 × 10	
	Hip adduction 2 × 10	
	Calf raise 2 × 10	
Abdominals (overload)	Weighted sit-up 3 × 4-7	
	Machine crunch 3 × 4-7	
Workout 6		
Chest (blood volume)	DB fly 4 × 14-20 superset with DB bench press 4 × 14-20	
	Pec dec 4 × 14-20 superset with hammer incline press 4 × 14-20	
Biceps (overload)	Barbell curl 3 × 4-7	
	Hammer curl 3 × 4-7	
	Machine preacher curl 3 × 4-7	
Triceps (overload)	Straight-bar cable pressdown 3 × 4-7	
	Skullcrusher 3 × 4-7	
	DB overhead extension 3 × 4-7	

Table 7.4   Sample Bikini Training Program: Weeks 1-3

	EXERCISE	WEEK 1	WEEK 2	WEEK 3
Day 1				
Back (L)	Deadlift	3 × 6	4 × 6	5 × 6
	Pendlay row	3 × 6-8	4 × 6-8	5 × 6-8
	Pull-up	2 × 6-8	3 × 6-8	4 × 6-8
	DB row	2 × 6-10	3 × 6-10	4 × 6-10
Glutes (M)	DB lunge	3-4 × 8-12/leg	3-4 × 8-12/leg	3-4 × 8-12/leg
	Hip thrust	2-4 × 10-12	2-4 × 10-12	2-4 × 10-12
	Weighted back extension	2-3 × 10-15	2-3 × 10-15	2-3 × 10-15
Abs	Cable crunch	2-4 × 10-15	2-4 × 10-15	2-4 × 10-15
Day 2				
Chest (M)	DB bench	2-4 × 8-12	2-4 × 8-12	2-4 × 8-12
Shoulders (M)	DB overhead press	2-4 × 10-12	2-4 × 10-12	2-4 × 10-12
	Seated side lateral raise	2-4 × 10-15	2-4 × 10-15	2-4 × 10-15
Arms (M)	Dip	2-4 × 8-12	2-4 × 8-12	2-4 × 8-12
	Standing EZ-bar curl	2-4 × 8-12	2-4 × 8-12	2-4 × 8-12
	Overhead cable extension	2-3 × 10-15	2-3 × 10-15	2-3 × 10-15
	Rope cable curl	2-3 × 10-15	2-3 × 10-15	2-3 × 10-15

	EXERCISE	WEEK 1	WEEK 2	WEEK 3
Day 3				
Lower body (L)	Squat	3 × 6	4 × 6	5 × 6
	RDL	3 × 6	4 × 6	5 × 6
	Leg extension	2 × 6-10	3 × 6-10	4 × 6-10
	Hamstring curl	2 × 6-10	3 × 6-10	4 × 6-10
Glutes (H)	Step back DB lunge	2-4 × 15-20	2-4 × 15-20	2-4 × 15-20
	Cable pull-through	2-4 × 15-25	2-4 × 15-25	2-4 × 15-25
	Banded hip thrust	2-4 × 20-30	2-4 × 20-30	2-4 × 20-30
Abs	Lying leg raise	2-4 × 10-15	2-4 × 10-15	2-4 × 10-15
Day 4				
Shoulders (L)	Barbell overhead press	3 × 6	4 × 6	5 × 6
	1-arm standing side lateral raise	3 × 6-10	4 × 6-10	5 × 6-10
	Upright row	2 × 6-10	3 × 6-10	4 × 6-10
	1-arm braced rear raise	2 × 6-10	3 × 6-10	4 × 6-10
Back (H)	Moto row	2-4 × 15-20	2-4 × 15-20	2-4 × 15-20
	Chest-supported row	2-4 × 15-20	2-4 × 15-20	2-4 × 15-20
	Straight-arm cable pressdown	2-3 × 20-30	2-3 × 20-30	2-3 × 20-30
Day 5				
Glutes (L)	Hip thrust	3 × 6	4 × 6	5 × 6
	Bulgarian split squat	3 × 6-8/leg	4 × 6-8/leg	5 × 6-8/leg
	Sumo leg press	2 × 6-10	3 × 6-10	4 × 6-10
Legs (H)	Hack squat	2-3 × 15-20	2-3 × 15-20	2-3 × 15-20
	Leg extension	2-3 × 20-30	2-3 × 20-30	2-3 × 20-30
	Hamstring curl	2-3 × 20-30	2-3 × 20-30	2-3 × 20-30
	Calf raise	2-4 × 15-25	2-4 × 15-25	2-4 × 15-25
Abs	Russian twist	2-4 × 8-12/side	2-4 × 8-12/side	2-4 × 8-12/side
Day 6				
Back (M)	Reverse-grip pulldown	3-4 × 8-12	3-4 × 8-12	3-4 × 8-12
	Meadows row	2-4 × 10-12	2-4 × 10-12	2-4 × 10-12
	Wide-grip cable row	2-3 × 10-15	2-3 × 10-15	2-3 × 10-15
Glutes (H)	Single-leg hip thrust	3-4 × 15-20	3-4 × 15-20	3-4 × 15-20
	Glute kickback	2-4 × 20-25	2-4 × 20-25	2-4 × 20-25
	Abductor machine	2-3 × 20-30	2-3 × 20-30	2-3 × 20-30
Shoulders (H)	Cable side lateral raise	4-6 × 20-30	4-6 × 20-30	4-6 × 20-30
Day 7				
Off day				

Table 7.5   Sample Bikini Training Program: Weeks 4-6

	EXERCISE	WEEK 4	WEEK 5	WEEK 6
Day 1				
Back (L)	Deadlift	3 × 5	4 × 5	5 × 5
	Pendlay row	3 × 5-7	4 × 5-7	5 × 5-7
	Pull-up	2 × 5-7	3 × 5-7	4 × 5-7
	DB row	2 × 6-8	3 × 6-8	4 × 6-8
Glutes (M)	DB lunge	3-4 × 6-10/leg	3-4 × 6-10/leg	3-4 × 6-10/leg
	Hip thrust	2-4 × 8-10	2-4 × 8-10	2-4 × 8-10
	Weighted back extension	2-3 × 8-12	2-3 × 8-12	2-3 × 8-12
Abs	Cable crunch	2-4 × 10-15	2-4 × 10-15	2-4 × 10-15
Day 2				
Chest (M)	DB bench	2-4 × 6-10	2-4 × 6-10	2-4 × 6-10
Shoulders (M)	DB overhead press	2-4 × 8-10	2-4 × 8-10	2-4 × 8-10
	Seated side lateral raise	2-4 × 8-12	2-4 × 8-12	2-4 × 8-12
Arms (M)	Dip	2-4 × 6-10	2-4 × 6-10	2-4 × 6-10
	Standing EZ-bar curl	2-4 × 6-10	2-4 × 6-10	2-4 × 6-10
	Overhead cable extension	2-3 × 8-12	2-3 × 8-12	2-3 × 8-12
	Rope cable curl	2-3 × 8-12	2-3 × 8-12	2-3 × 8-12
Day 3				
Lower body (L)	Squat	3 × 5	4 × 5	5 × 5
	RDL	3 × 5	4 × 5	5 × 5
	Leg extension	2 × 6-8	3 × 6-8	4 × 6-8
	Hamstring curl	2 × 6-8	3 × 6-8	4 × 6-8
Glutes (H)	Step back DB lunge	2-4 × 15-20	2-4 × 15-20	2-4 × 15-20
	Cable pull-through	2-4 × 15-25	2-4 × 15-25	2-4 × 15-25
	Banded hip thrust	2-4 × 20-30	2-4 × 20-30	2-4 × 20-30
Abs	Lying leg raise	2-4 × 10-15	2-4 × 10-15	2-4 × 10-15
Day 4				
Shoulders (L)	Barbell overhead press	3 × 5	4 × 5	5 × 5
	1-arm standing side lateral raise	3 × 6-8	4 × 6-8	5 × 6-8
	Upright row	2 × 6-8	3 × 6-8	4 × 6-8
	1-arm braced rear raise	2 × 6-8	3 × 6-8	4 × 6-8
Back (H)	Moto row	2-4 × 15-20	2-4 × 15-20	2-4 × 15-20
	Chest-supported row	2-4 × 15-20	2-4 × 15-20	2-4 × 15-20
	Straight-arm cable pressdown	2-3 × 20-30	2-3 × 20-30	2-3 × 20-30
Day 5				
Glutes (L)	Hip thrust	3 × 5	4 × 5	5 × 5

	EXERCISE	WEEK 4	WEEK 5	WEEK 6
	Bulgarian split squat	3 × 5-7/leg	4 × 5-7/leg	5 × 5-7/leg
	Sumo leg press	2 × 6-8	3 × 6-8	4 × 6-8
Legs (H)	Hack squat	2-3 × 15-20	2-3 × 15-20	2-3 × 15-20
	Leg extension	2-3 × 20-30	2-3 × 20-30	2-3 × 20-30
	Hamstring curl	2-3 × 20-30	2-3 × 20-30	2-3 × 20-30
	Calf raise	2-4 × 15-25	2-4 × 15-25	2-4 × 15-25
Abs	Russian twist	2-4 × 8-12/side	2-4 × 8-12/side	2-4 × 8-12/side
Day 6				
Back (M)	Reverse-grip pulldown	3-4 × 6-10	3-4 × 6-10	3-4 × 6-10
	Meadows row	2-4 × 8-10	2-4 × 8-10	2-4 × 8-10
	Wide-grip cable row	2-3 × 8-12	2-3 × 8-12	2-3 × 8-12
Glutes (H)	Single-leg hip thrust	3-4 × 15-20	3-4 × 15-20	3-4 × 15-20
	Glute kickback	2-4 × 20-25	2-4 × 20-25	2-4 × 20-25
	Abductor machine	2-3 × 20-30	2-3 × 20-30	2-3 × 20-30
Shoulders (H)	Cable side lateral raise	4-6 × 20-30	4-6 × 20-30	4-6 × 20-30
Day 7				
Off day				

Table 7.6 Sample Bikini Training Program: Weeks 7-9

	EXERCISE	WEEK 7	WEEK 8	WEEK 9
Day 1				
Back (L)	Deadlift	3 × 4	4 × 4	5 × 4
	Pendlay row	3 × 4-6	4 × 4-6	5 × 4-6
	Pull-up	2 × 4-6	3 × 4-6	4 × 4-6
	DB row	2 × 5-8	3 × 5-8	4 × 5-8
Glutes (M)	DB lunge	3-4 × 6-8/leg	3-4 × 6-8/leg	3-4 × 6-8/leg
	Hip thrust	2-4 × 6-10	2-4 × 6-10	2-4 × 6-10
	Weighted back extension	2-3 × 8-10	2-3 × 8-10	2-3 × 8-10
Abs	Cable crunch	2-4 × 10-15	2-4 × 10-15	2-4 × 10-15
Day 2				
Chest (M)	DB bench	2-4 × 6-8	2-4 × 6-8	2-4 × 6-8
Shoulders (M)	DB overhead press	2-4 × 6-10	2-4 × 6-10	2-4 × 6-10
	Seated side lateral raise	2-4 × 8-10	2-4 × 8-10	2-4 × 8-10
Arms (M)	Dip	2-4 × 6-8	2-4 × 6-8	2-4 × 6-8
	Standing EZ-bar curl	2-4 × 6-8	2-4 × 6-8	2-4 × 6-8
	Overhead cable extension	2-3 × 8-10	2-3 × 8-10	2-3 × 8-10
	Rope cable curl	2-3 × 8-10	2-3 × 8-10	2-3 × 8-10

(continued)

Table 7.6 *(continued)*

	EXERCISE	WEEK 7	WEEK 8	WEEK 9
Day 3				
Lower body (L)	Squat	3 × 4	4 × 4	5 × 4
	RDL	3 × 4	4 × 4	5 × 4
	Leg extension	2 × 5-8	3 × 5-8	4 × 5-8
	Hamstring curl	2 × 5-8	3 × 5-8	4 × 5-8
Glutes (H)	Step back DB lunge	2-4 × 15-20	2-4 × 15-20	2-4 × 15-20
	Cable pull-through	2-4 × 15-25	2-4 × 15-25	2-4 × 15-25
	Banded hip thrust	2-4 × 20-30	2-4 × 20-30	2-4 × 20-30
Abs	Lying leg raise	2-4 × 10-15	2-4 × 10-15	2-4 × 10-15
Day 4				
Shoulders (L)	Barbell overhead press	3 × 4	4 × 4	5 × 4
	1-arm standing side lateral raise	3 × 5-8	4 × 5-8	5 × 5-8
	Upright row	2 × 5-8	3 × 5-8	4 × 5-8
	1-arm braced rear raise	2 × 5-8	3 × 5-8	4 × 5-8
Back (H)	Moto row	2-4 × 15-20	2-4 × 15-20	2-4 × 15-20
	Chest-supported row	2-4 × 15-20	2-4 × 15-20	2-4 × 15-20
	Straight-arm cable pressdown	2-3 × 20-30	2-3 × 20-30	2-3 × 20-30
Day 5				
Glutes (L)	Hip thrust	3 × 4	4 × 4	5 × 4
	Bulgarian split squat	3 × 4-6/leg	4 × 4-7/leg	5 × 4-7/leg
	Sumo leg press	2 × 5-8	3 × 5-8	4 × 5-8
Legs (H)	Hack squat	2-3 × 15-20	2-3 × 15-20	2-3 × 15-20
	Leg extension	2-3 × 20-30	2-3 × 20-30	2-3 × 20-30
	Hamstring curl	2-3 × 20-30	2-3 × 20-30	2-3 × 20-30
	Calf raise	2-4 × 15-25	2-4 × 15-25	2-4 × 15-25
Abs	Russian twist	2-4 × 8-12/side	2-4 × 8-12/side	2-4 × 8-12/side
Day 6				
Back (M)	Reverse-grip pulldown	3-4 × 6-8	3-4 × 6-8	3-4 × 6-8
	Meadows row	2-4 × 6-10	2-4 × 6-10	2-4 × 6-10
	Wide-grip cable row	2-3 × 8-10	2-3 × 8-10	2-3 × 8-10
Glutes (H)	Single-leg hip thrust	3-4 × 15-20	3-4 × 15-20	3-4 × 15-20
	Glute kickback	2-4 × 20-25	2-4 × 20-25	2-4 × 20-25
	Abductor machine	2-3 × 20-30	2-3 × 20-30	2-3 × 20-30
Shoulders (H)	Cable side lateral raise	4-6 × 20-30	4-6 × 20-30	4-6 × 20-30
Day 7				
Off day				

Take-Home Points

► Increasing exercise and nonexercise activity can create an energy deficit. However, try to perform as little formal cardio as possible while still achieving your target rate of weight loss. Base the intensity of cardio on your recovery ability and preexisting injury history.

► Tracking step counts during contest prep can keep you active during daily life and help prevent a decline in energy expenditure outside the gym.

► Maintaining training intensity through contest prep is key for muscle preservation. Continue to focus on progressive overload throughout contest prep.

► Increasing training volume results in increased muscle growth if you do not exceed your recovery ability. Allocating this volume into two or three workouts weekly may result in more progress than training body parts once weekly.

► There is no "best" repetition range for muscle growth. Training throughout a variety of repetition ranges may be superior for muscle growth than consistently performing the same number of reps.

► Take deload weeks and extra days off from the gym as necessary for recovery. There is no award for pushing through when you are feeling beat down. If anything, you will slow progression and increase injury risk.

► You should do a workout you enjoy in the gym as long as it is reasonable for your goals. If you enjoy what you are doing, you are likely to work harder, stay more consistent, and see more progress.

The Art of Posing

Bodybuilding has long been viewed as a combination of art and science. Posing is more the artistic side of the sport. Beginners and advanced competitors alike often misunderstand it. When most competitors think of posing, they quickly get the image of squeezing and flexing as hard as they can onstage to show muscularity and conditioning. While this is indeed part of posing, the main component of effective posing is displaying your body effectively. The judges can only judge what they can see. You can win or lose a show depending on how you display your physique. Years of training and months of dieting may all be for nothing if you do not display your physique to its fullest potential.

Attend any bodybuilding show, and you will quickly see who did his or her homework when it comes to posing. When competitors walk out onstage, it is not uncommon for some of them to look impressive while others look average. As they begin to pose, some competitors' physiques will practically pop off the stage, and others seem to fade. This is almost always due to effective posing execution.

In this section, we will cover all the dos and don'ts of effective posing as well as the way to efficiently practice and prepare for posing come show day.

Pose Finder

DIVISION AND POSE NAME	PAGE NUMBER
Bodybuilding (men and women)	
Front standing relaxed	96
Side standing relaxed	98
Rear standing relaxed	100
Front double biceps	102
Front lat spread	104
Side chest	106
Side triceps	108
Back (or rear) double biceps	110
Back (or rear) lat spread	112
Hands overhead abdominal (or ab and thigh)	114
Hands on hips most muscular	116
Crab most muscular	118
Hands clasped most muscular	120
Classic physique (men)	
Front standing relaxed	122
Side standing relaxed	124
Rear standing relaxed	126
Front double biceps	128
Side chest	130
Back (or rear) double biceps	132
Hands overhead abdominal (or ab and thigh)	134
Favorite classic pose	136
Men's physique	
Front pose	138
Side pose	140
Back pose	142
Women's physique	
Front standing relaxed	144
Side standing relaxed	146
Rear standing relaxed	148
Front double biceps	150
Side chest with leg extended	152
Side triceps with leg extended	154

DIVISION AND POSE NAME	PAGE NUMBER
Women's physique	
Back (or rear) double biceps	156
Hands overhead abdominal (or ab and thigh)	158
Figure (women)	
Front pose	160
Side pose	162
Back pose	164
Bikini (women)	
Front pose	166
Back pose	168

BODYBUILDING (MEN AND WOMEN)

Men and women who compete in the bodybuilding division have two rounds of judging: the standing relaxed poses and the mandatory poses.

Round 1: Standing Relaxed Poses

At prejudging, you will be judged first on the **standing relaxed poses**. Do not let the name deceive you; there is nothing relaxing about them! Back when bodybuilding first started, the judges indeed wanted to view the competitors in a relaxed pose. Inevitably, some competitors would try to flex a bit to give themselves an advantage. Over the years, judges allowed more flexing in the standing relaxed round, and today they expect it.

▶ Front standing relaxed • Side standing relaxed • Rear standing relaxed

Round 2: Mandatory Poses

After the standing relaxed poses, the judges will have you face the front once again. This is when they prepare for the mandatory poses and call out specific poses. You and the other competitors execute the poses until the judge says to relax. Then go into your relaxed pose from the first round. At no point on stage should you ever actually relax and not pose.

▶ Front double biceps • Front lat spread • Side chest • Side triceps • Back (or rear) double biceps • Back (or rear) lat spread • Hands overhead abdominal (or ab and thigh)

Most Muscular

The final pose is the most muscular pose. A most muscular pose can be performed multiple ways, and we will touch on each one.

▶ Hands on hips most muscular • Crab most muscular • Hands clasped most muscular

CLASSIC PHYSIQUE (MEN)

Men who compete in the classic physique division have two rounds of judging, like the men's and women's bodybuilding divisions.

Round 1: Standing Relaxed Poses

At prejudging, you will be judged first on the standing relaxed poses. Do not let the name deceive you; there is nothing relaxing about them! Back when bodybuilding first started, the judges indeed wanted to view the competitors in a relaxed pose. Inevitably, some competitors would try to flex a bit to give themselves an advantage. Over the years, judges allowed more flexing in the standing relaxed round, and today they expect it.

▶ Front standing relaxed · Side standing relaxed · Rear standing relaxed

Round 2: Mandatory Poses

After the standing relaxed poses, the judges will have you face the front once again. This is when they prepare for the mandatory poses. In this round, they call out specific poses. You and all other competitors execute the poses until the judge says to relax. Then go into the relaxed pose again from the first round. At no point on stage should you ever actually relax and not pose.

▶ Front double biceps · Side chest · Back (or rear) double biceps · Hands overhead abdominal (or ab and thigh) · Favorite classic pose

MEN'S PHYSIQUE

The men's physique division has far fewer poses than bodybuilding or classic physique. As discussed previously, this also means you have fewer ways to beat your opponents than in bodybuilding or classic physique.

Quarter Turns

In this division, you only have one round of comparison poses, but you will be put through each pose several times using quarter turns.

▶ Front pose · Side pose · Back pose

WOMEN'S PHYSIQUE

Like the men's classic physique division, the women's physique division has two rounds of judging and versions of several poses specific to the division.

Round 1: Standing Relaxed Poses

At prejudging, you will be judged first on the standing relaxed poses. Do not let the name deceive you; there is nothing relaxing about them! Back when bodybuilding first started, the judges indeed wanted to view the competitors in a relaxed pose. Inevitably, some competitors would try to flex a bit to give themselves an advantage. Over the years, judges allowed more flexing in the standing relaxed round, and today, they expect it.

▶ Front standing relaxed · Side standing relaxed · Rear standing relaxed

Round 2: Mandatory Poses

After the standing relaxed poses, the judges will have you face the front once again. This is when they prepare for the mandatory poses. In this round, they call out specific poses. You and all other competitors execute the poses until the judge says to relax. Then go into the relaxed pose again from the first round. At no point onstage should you ever actually relax and not pose.

▶ Front double biceps • Side chest with leg extended • Side triceps with leg extended • Back (or rear) double biceps • Hands overhead abdominal (or ab and thigh)

FIGURE (WOMEN)

Much like the men's physique division, women's figure has fewer poses than bodybuilding or women's physique. In this division, you only have one round of comparison poses, but you will be put through each pose several times.

▶ Front pose • Side pose • Back pose

BIKINI (WOMEN)

Bikini posing is quite different compared to other divisions. The other divisions have quarter turns, but bikini only uses half turns. While there are fewer poses, and the poses are seemingly less difficult to execute, the subtlety of bikini posing should be considered carefully. In this division, being able to pose and make it look natural as well as effortless counts for a lot. Practice should not be taken lightly.

One final note: While divisions can have slightly different criteria for posing depending on which federation you compete in, bikini probably has the most variation between competing sanctions. For this reason, check the guidelines for the specific federation you are competing in.

▶ Front pose • Back pose

FRONT STANDING RELAXED

When you first walk out on stage with the other competitors, you will be lined up, and you should immediately execute the front standing relaxed pose. The judges will not call out this pose because you are expected to go directly into it.

To properly perform a front standing relaxed pose, face the judges. When executing any pose, run through a checklist of where your body parts should be from the ground up. As you face the

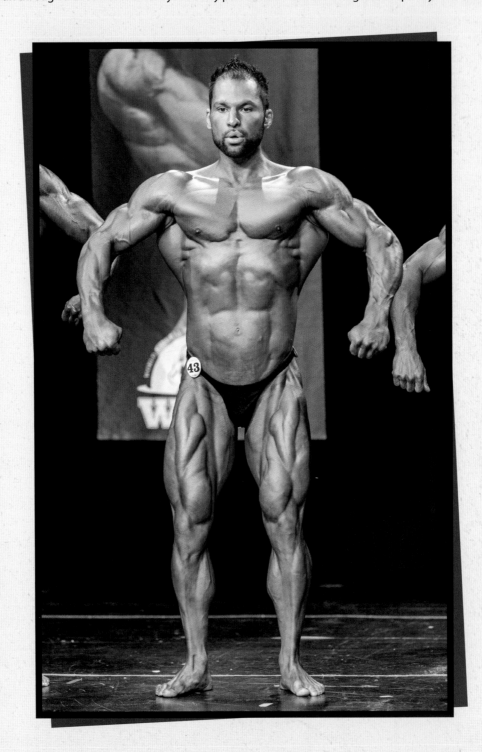

judges, set your feet just a bit narrower than shoulder width, with your toes slightly turned outward to enhance quadriceps sweep. Flex your quads by pushing your feet against the ground, almost as if you were trying push your feet through the floor. Shift your hips back ever so slightly to cause separation in your upper quads. Next, raise your ribcage as high as you can and pull your abdominal wall in as far as you can. Imagine trying to touch your navel to your spine. Flare your lats and keep your arms out at your sides at roughly a 45-degree angle. Keep your shoulder girdle down, keep your chin up, and aim to have a relaxed facial expression in all your poses.

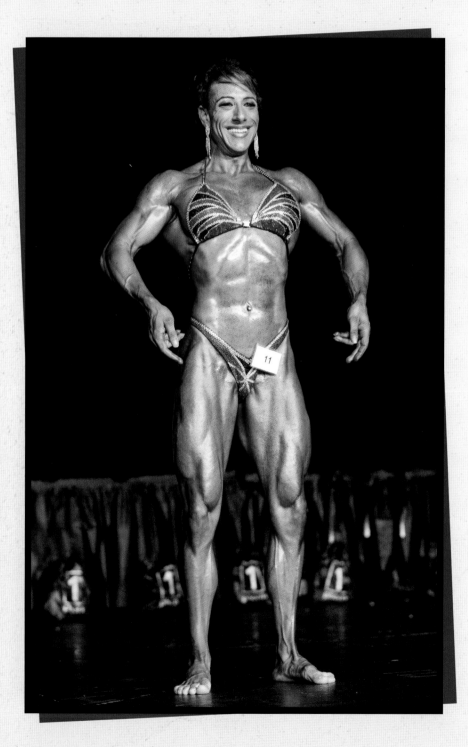

SIDE STANDING RELAXED

After the front standing relaxed pose, the judges will say, "Quarter turn." Always turn to the right. Then go directly into the side standing relaxed pose.

Start the side standing relaxed pose by facing the side of the stage. Your feet should be touching or almost touching, with the foot closest to the judges about one or two inches

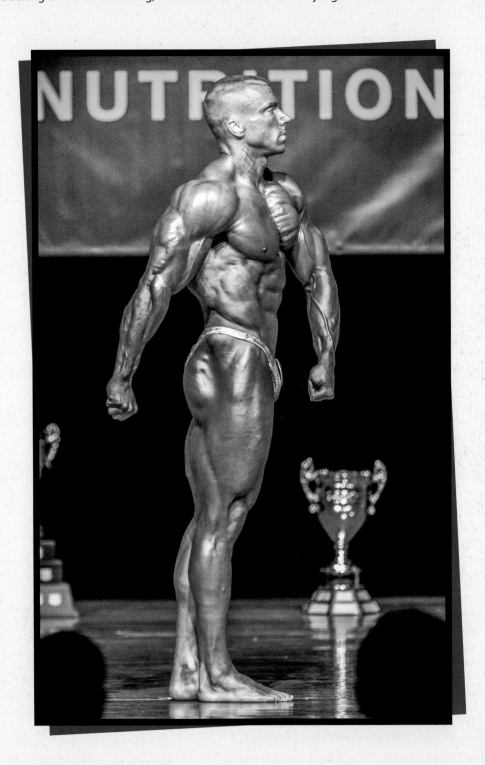

(2.5-5 cm) in front of the other foot. Slightly bend the knee closest to the judges and flex your glutes. Keeping your rib cage down or in a neutral position, flex your abs, and pull your abdominal wall in as far as you possibly can. Flex your pecs and turn your shoulders very slightly to open up to the judges. Use your back arm to slightly push into your back pectoral. Keep your chin up and your head facing to the side of the stage. Do not look at the judges during the side standing relaxed pose.

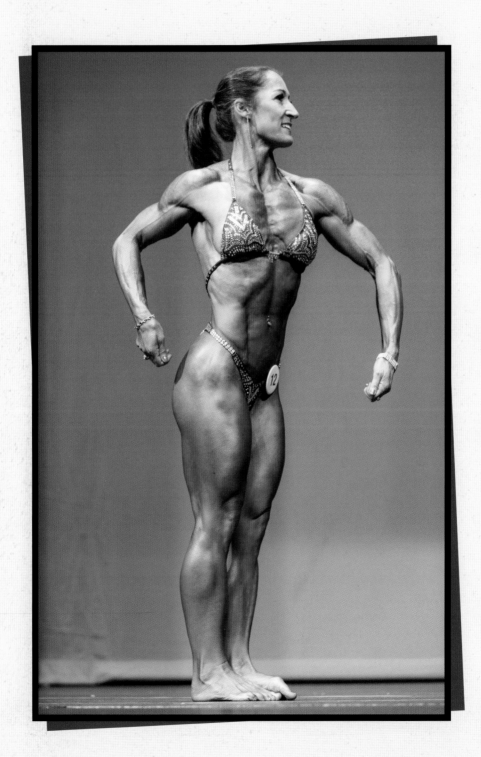

REAR STANDING RELAXED

After the side standing relaxed, the judges will again say, "Quarter turn to the right." You should then face the back of the stage with your back toward the judges and go directly into the rear standing relaxed pose. Start with your feet just narrower than shoulder width. Turn your toes slightly out to the sides so that your outer quads are visible from the back. Bend your

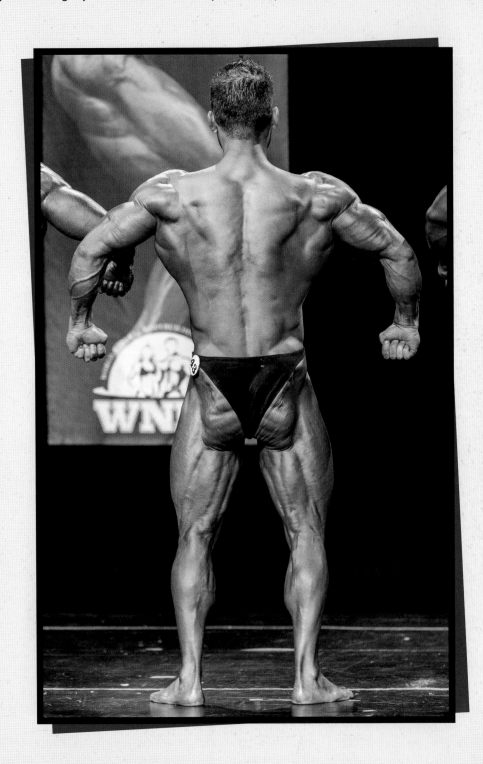

knees a little and flex your hamstrings by imagining pressing your heels backward. You should then squeeze and flex your glutes very tightly. Flare and flex your lats as you bring your arms to your sides at roughly a 45-degree angle. Lean back ever so slightly and keep your head up.

After your rear standing relaxed, the judges will once again say, "Quarter turn." At this point, you perform your side standing relaxed pose while facing the other direction.

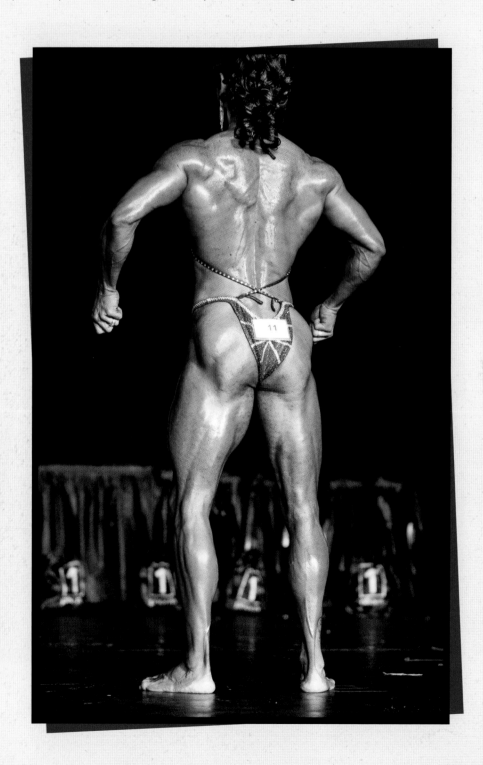

FRONT DOUBLE BICEPS

The front double biceps pose is often called first in the mandatory posing round. You can set your feet in one of two ways. You may either keep your feet stationary as they are in the front standing relaxed pose, or you may bring one leg forward to display the quad. Pull your

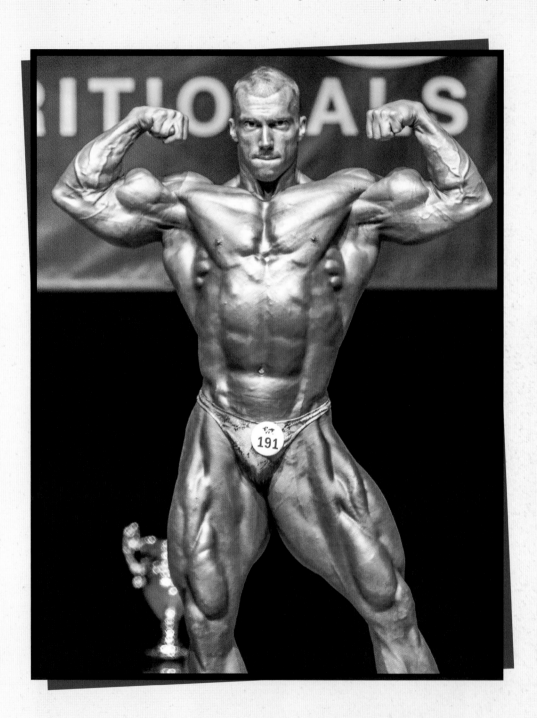

ribcage up as you pull in your abdominal wall as far as you can. Raise your arms, with your elbows just slightly in front of your torso, and flex your biceps. Keep your chin up and your shoulders down.

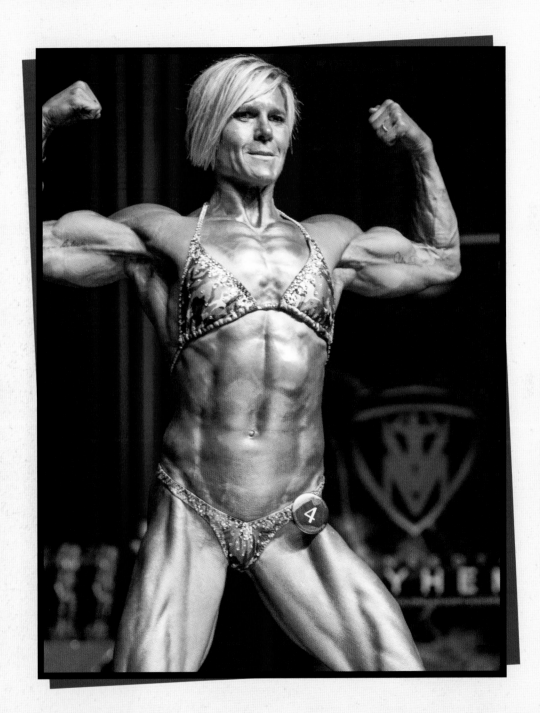

FRONT LAT SPREAD

The front lat spread should begin with your feet set as they are in your front standing relaxed pose. Flex your quads, and shift your hips back. Pull your ribcage upward and pull your abdomen in. Place your hands at your sides just above your hips, with your fists in a

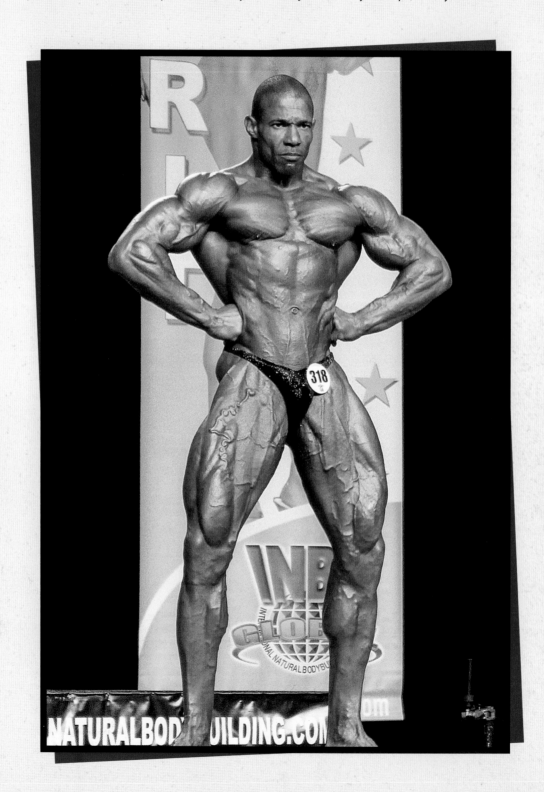

ball. Flare your lats as widely as you can. Keep your chest up, shoulders down, and chin up. A common mistake in this pose is trying to flex your lats. However, the lats do not need to be flexed, only flared.

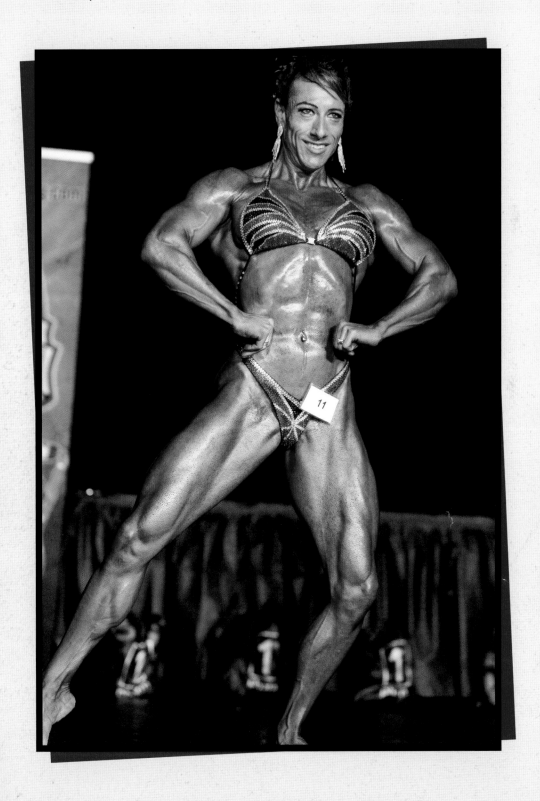

SIDE CHEST

After the front double biceps and front lat spread poses, the judges will ask you to quarter turn and face the side. The first pose usually called is the side chest pose. In this pose, you spike the calf closest to the judges by bringing your heel off of the ground and shifting your weight onto your toes. Then squat down slightly: Your thigh should be about a 35- to 55-de-

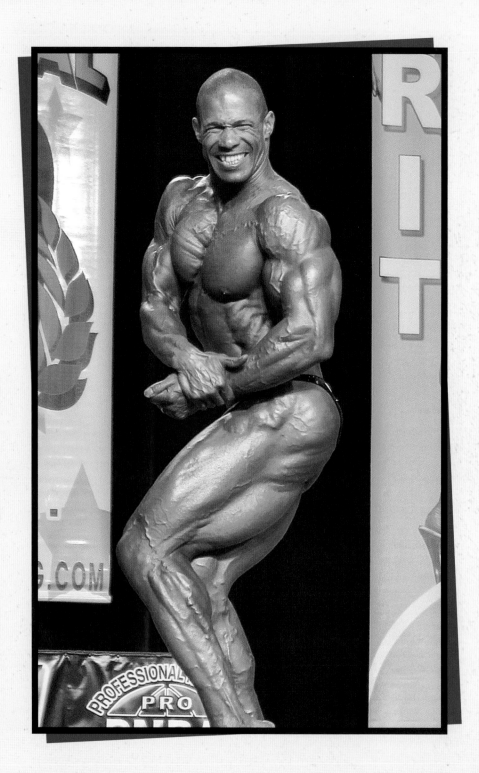

gree angle to the floor. Take the knee furthest from the judges and push it slightly into your other leg. Flex the hamstring and glute closest to the judges. Place your ribcage in a neutral position while you flex your abs and intercostals and pull your abdomen inward as far as you can. Clasp your hands in front of you and flex your pecs as you twist your torso ever so slightly toward the judges. Keep your shoulder down and your chin up.

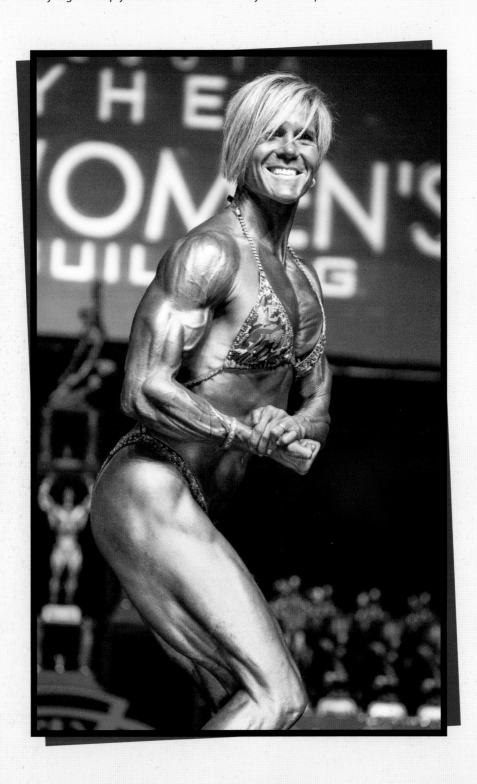

SIDE TRICEPS

The side triceps pose begins with your feet and legs set just as they are in the side chest pose. However, instead of clasping your hands in front, clasp them behind your back. You can do this by either locking your fingers together or using your back hand to grab the wrist of your front hand. Keep your torso in an upright position as you flex your abs and intercos-

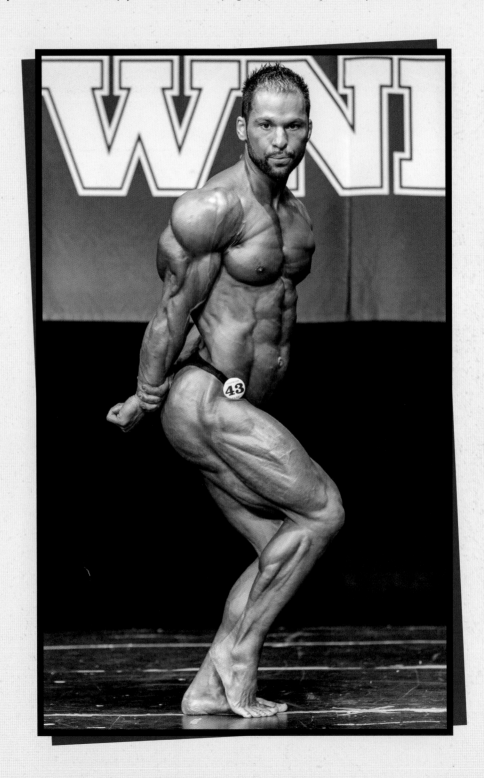

tals while pulling your abdominal wall in as far as you can. Open your body ever so slightly toward the judges but do not pull your arm behind you. Your goal should be to display the triceps prominently to the judges. Do not shrug your shoulders; this is a common mistake. Keep your chin up.

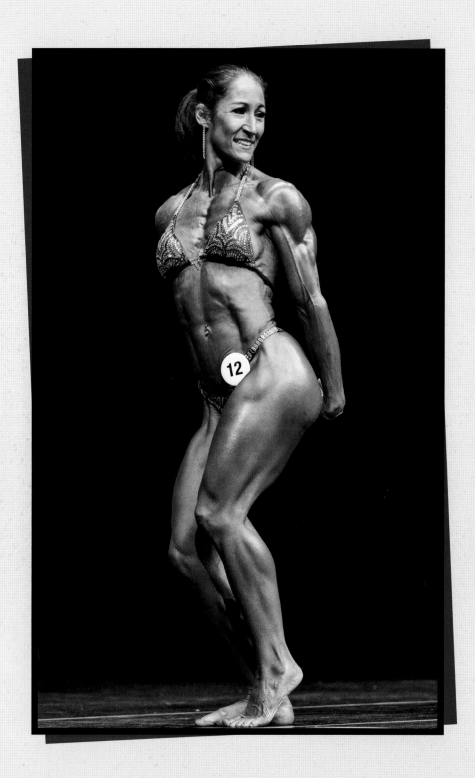

BACK (OR REAR) DOUBLE BICEPS

After you complete the side mandatory poses, the judges will have you quarter turn toward the back of the stage. Typically, they will call out *rear double biceps pose*, sometimes called the *back double biceps pose*. Place one foot behind you and spike your calf. Sometimes the judges specify which calf you should spike. If they do not specify which foot to place behind, then pick the one you feel most comfortable with. Place your foot behind your other foot approx-

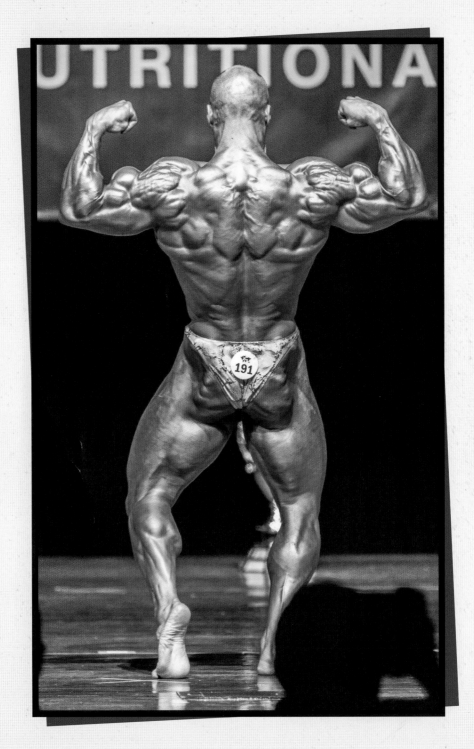

imately 10 to 15 inches (25-38 cm). Your knees should be turned outward slightly and bent just a little. Flex both hamstrings by digging your feet against the floor, as if you were trying to perform a leg curl. Flex and squeeze your glutes tightly. Bring your arms out to your sides and flex your biceps and the entire muscularity of your back. You should not pinch your shoulder blades together. Instead, keep them open so that your back stays wide. Lean your torso back ever so slightly toward the judges.

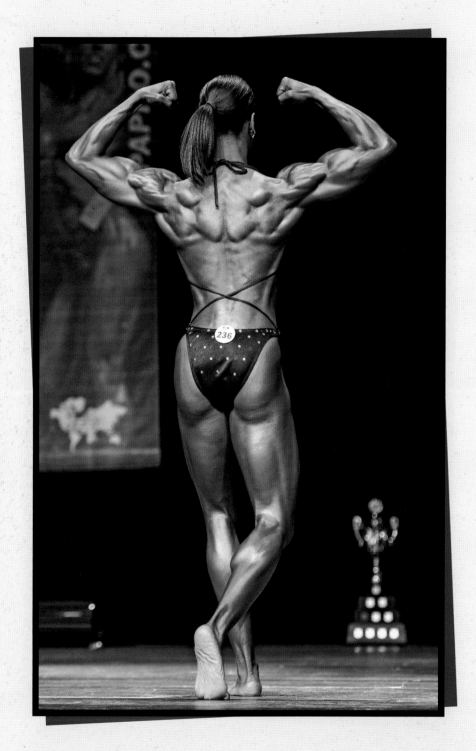

BACK (OR REAR) LAT SPREAD

The rear lat spread, sometimes called the *back lat spread*, begins with the same leg position as the back double biceps pose. Place one foot behind you and spike the calf. Sometimes the judges specify which calf you should spike. If they do not specify which foot to place behind, then pick the one you feel most comfortable with. Place your foot behind your other foot approximately 10 to 15 inches (25-38 cm). Your knees should be turned outward slightly and

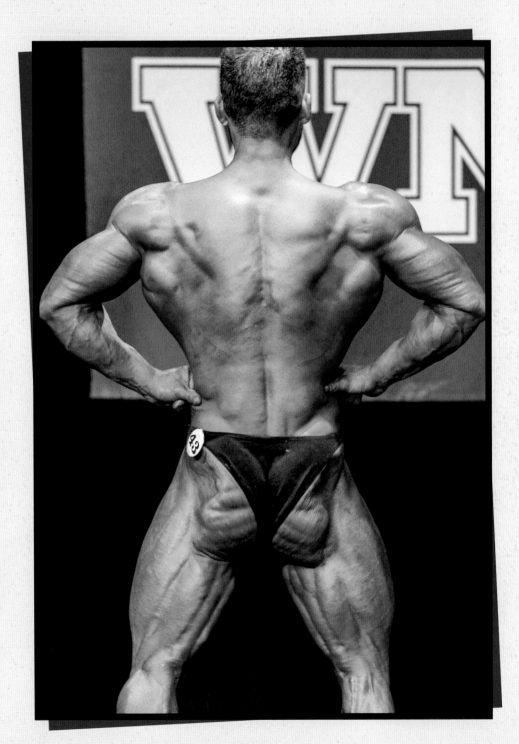

bent just a little. Flex both hamstrings by digging your feet against the floor, as if you were trying to perform a leg curl. Flex and squeeze your glutes tightly. You should lean back ever so slightly as you place your hands on your sides just above your hips and hook your thumbs. Open up your shoulder blades and flare your lats. Keep your chest high. On this pose, you flex your lats, as opposed to the front lat spread, where you do not need to flex the lats. Keep your shoulders down and do not shrug because this diminishes the muscularity in your back. Keep your chin up.

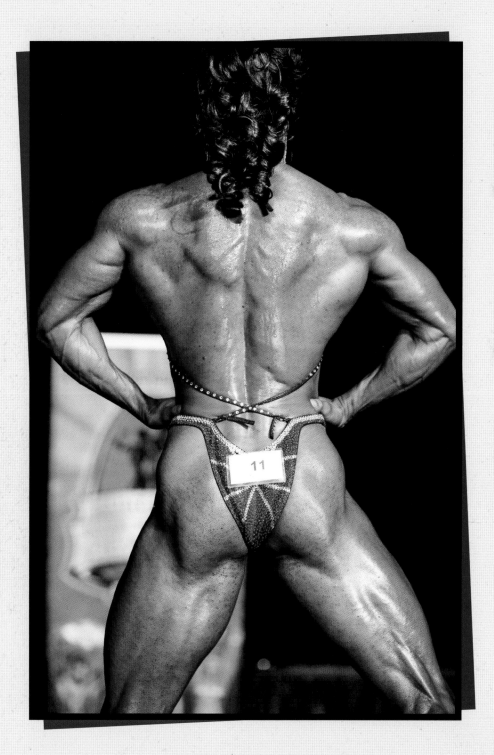

HANDS OVERHEAD ABDOMINAL (OR AB AND THIGH)

After the back poses, the judges may have you perform the side chest and side triceps poses on the other side. Then they will bring you back around to the front for the hands overhead

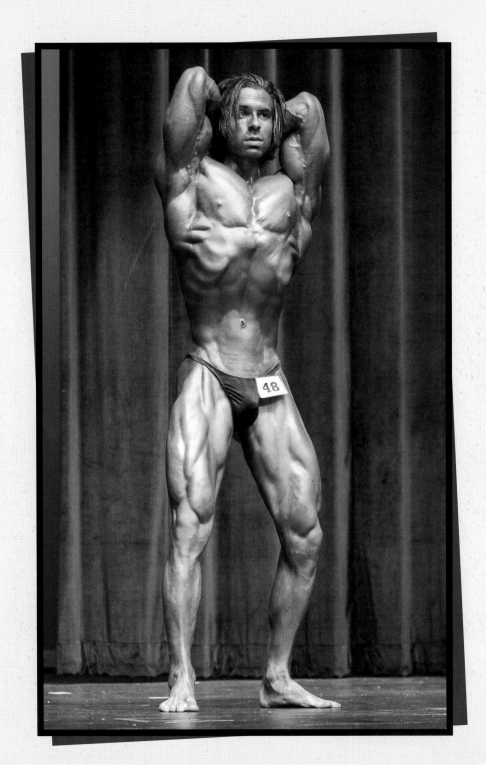

abdominal pose. This pose is also sometimes called the *ab and thigh pose*. Begin this pose by placing one leg in front of the other and spiking the calf. Sometimes judges specify which leg they want to see. If they do not specify which leg to place forward, then use the leg you are most comfortable with. Flex the quads in both legs, but make sure you prominently display the quads on the forward leg. Raise your hands and place them behind your head. Then flex your abs as hard as you can while you slightly crunch down to increase the contraction. Keep your pecs and arms flexed and your arms as close as possible to your head.

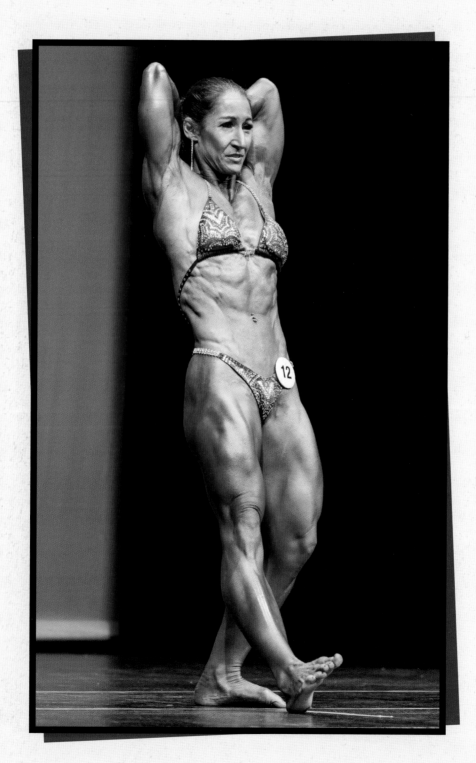

HANDS ON HIPS MOST MUSCULAR

With the hands on hips most muscular, begin by setting your legs just as you would in a front standing relaxed pose, with your hips back and quads flexed. Keep your ribcage down as you flex your abs. Bring your hands to your sides and flex your pecs and arms

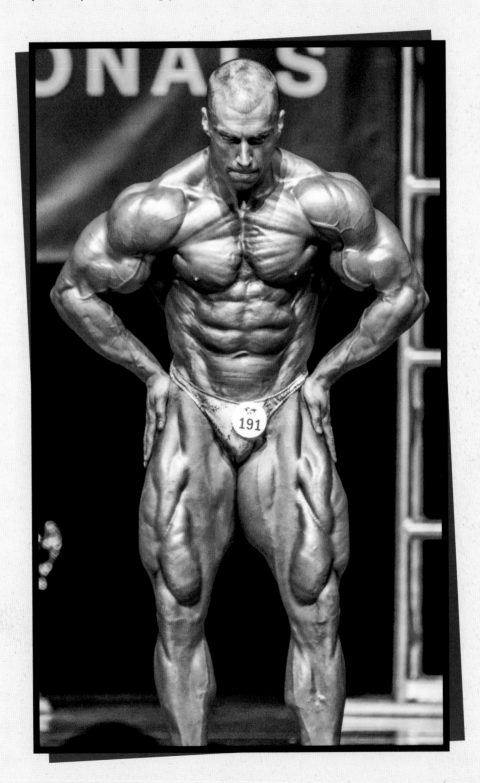

by pressing into your hips hard. Keep your shoulders down and chin up. This type of most muscular pose tends to look good on those with great shape or great shoulder development.

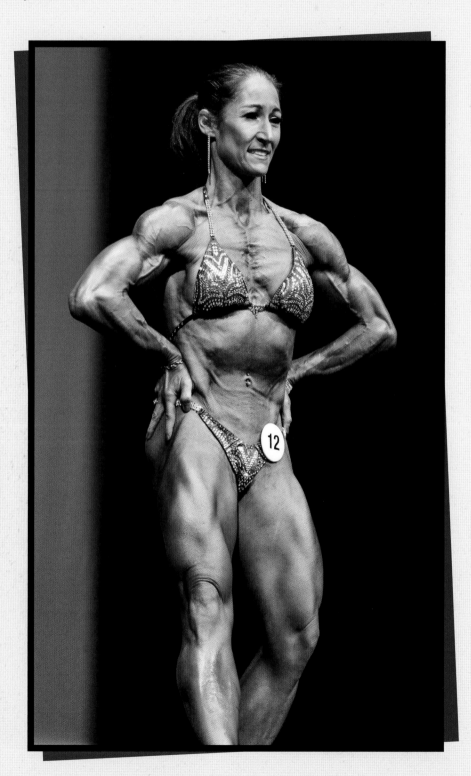

CRAB MOST MUSCULAR

The crab most muscular is the pose that most people think of when they think of a "most muscular" pose. In this version, you place one leg forward and flex your quad. Inhale as much air as possible while raising your ribcage and pulling your abs in. Lean over slightly as you bring

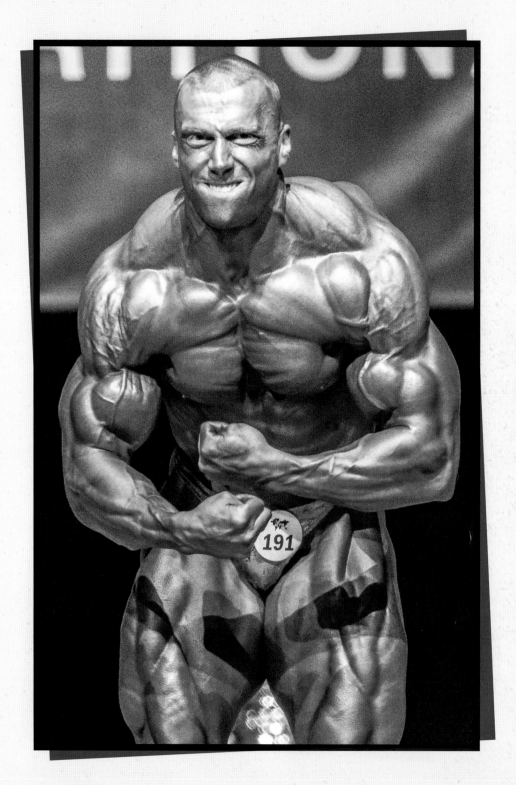

your arms in front of your body and flex your biceps, shoulders, traps, and pecs all at once. This type of most muscular pose tends to look great on those with good overall muscle size in the chest, traps, and arms.

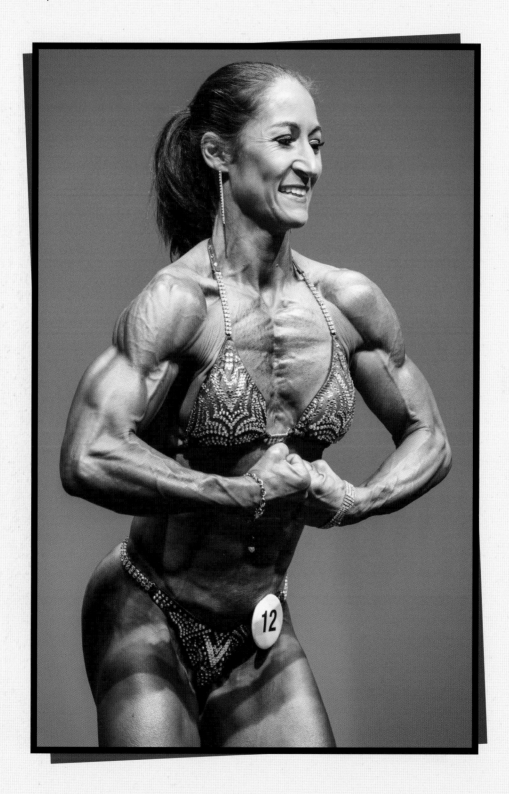

HANDS CLASPED MOST MUSCULAR

The hands clasped most muscular begins with your legs set just as they are in a front standing relaxed pose. With your ribcage in a neutral position, flex your abs and pull your abdominal wall in. Bring your hands to the front and clasp them together. Push your hands together to

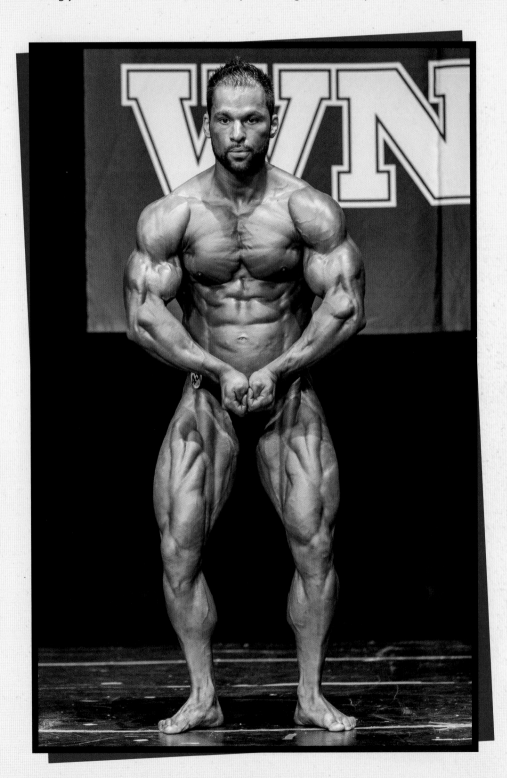

flex your arms, pecs, and shoulders. Be careful not to pinch your shoulders inward because it can make you look narrow and smaller. This most muscular pose tends to look good on very lean competitors because it prominently shows off the conditioning of all parts of the body.

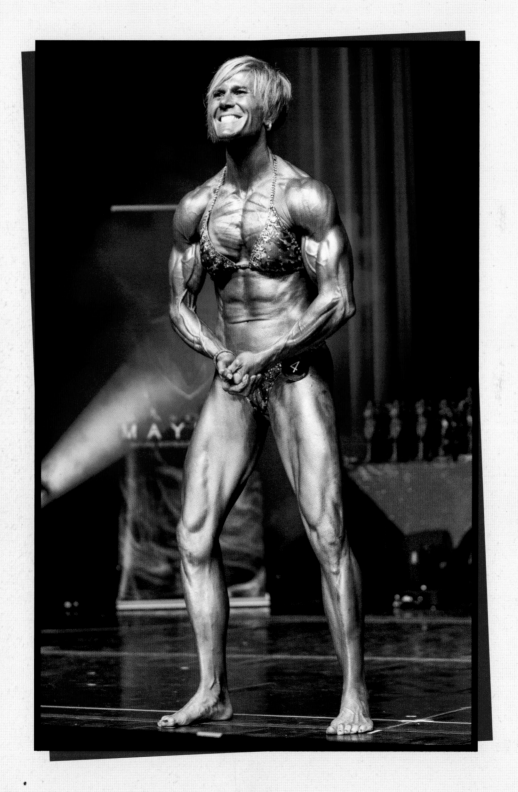

FRONT STANDING RELAXED

When you first walk out onstage with the other competitors, you will be lined up, and you should immediately do the front standing relaxed pose. The judges will not call out this pose because you are expected to go directly into it.

To properly perform a front standing relaxed pose, face the judges. When executing any pose, run through a checklist of where your body parts should be from the ground up. As you face the judges, set your feet just a bit narrower than shoulder width, with your toes slightly turned outward to enhance quad sweep. Flex your quads, pushing your feet against the ground, almost as if you were trying push your feet through the floor. Shift your hips back ever so slightly so they cause separation in your upper quads. Next, raise your ribcage as high as you can and pull your abdominal wall in as far as you can. Imagine trying to touch your navel to your spine. Flare your lats and keep your arms out at your sides at roughly a 45-degree angle. Keep your shoulder girdle down, keep your chin up, and aim to have a relaxed facial expression in all your poses.

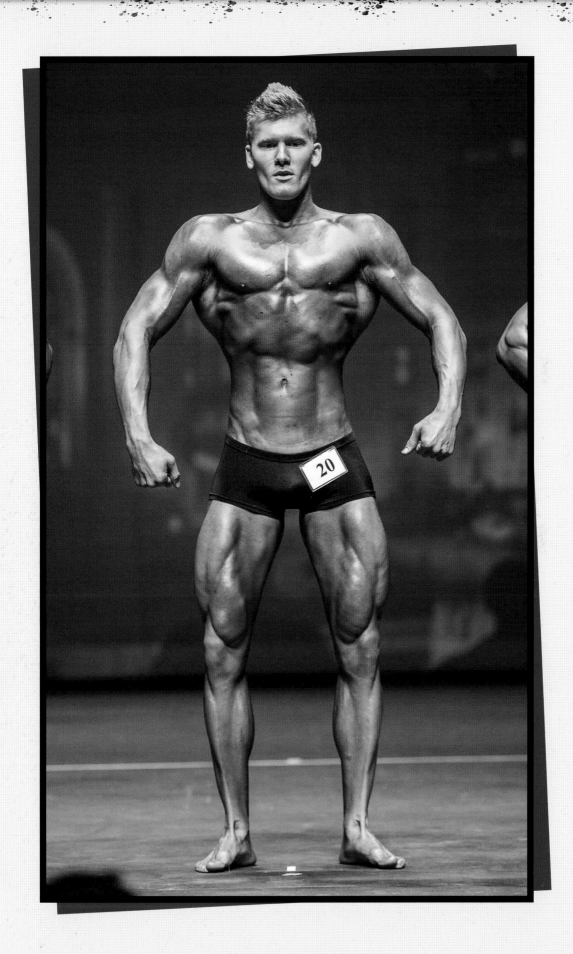

SIDE STANDING RELAXED

After the front standing relaxed pose, the judges will say, "Quarter turn." Always turn to the right. Then go directly into the side standing relaxed pose.

Start the side standing relaxed pose by facing the side of the stage. Your feet should be touching or almost touching, with the foot closest to the judges about one or two inches (2.5-5 cm) in front of the other foot. Slightly bend the knee closest to the judges. Keeping your rib cage down or in a neutral position, flex your abs and pull your abdominal wall in as far as you possibly can. Flex your pecs and turn your shoulders very slightly to open up to the judges. Use your back arm to slightly push into your back pectoral. Keep your chin up and keep your head facing to the side of the stage. Do not look at the judges while in the side standing relaxed pose.

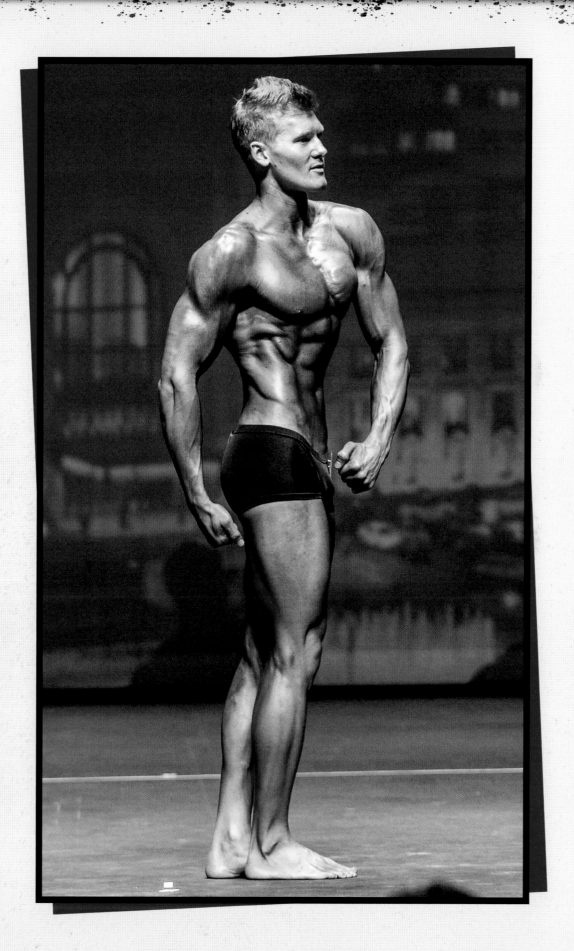

REAR STANDING RELAXED

After the side standing relaxed, the judges will say, "Quarter turn to the right." You should face the back of the stage, with your back toward the judges. You will go directly into the rear standing relaxed pose. Start with your feet just narrower than shoulder width. Turn your toes slightly out to the sides so that your outer quads are visible from the back. Bend your knees a little and flex your hamstrings by imagining pressing your heels backward. You should then squeeze your glutes, but there is no need to do so very tightly because they are not visible in classic physique. Flare and flex your lats as you bring your arms to your sides at roughly a 45-degree angle. Lean back ever so slightly and keep your head up.

After your rear standing relaxed, the judges will once again say, "Quarter turn." You will face the other side. At this point, perform your side standing relaxed pose while facing the other direction.

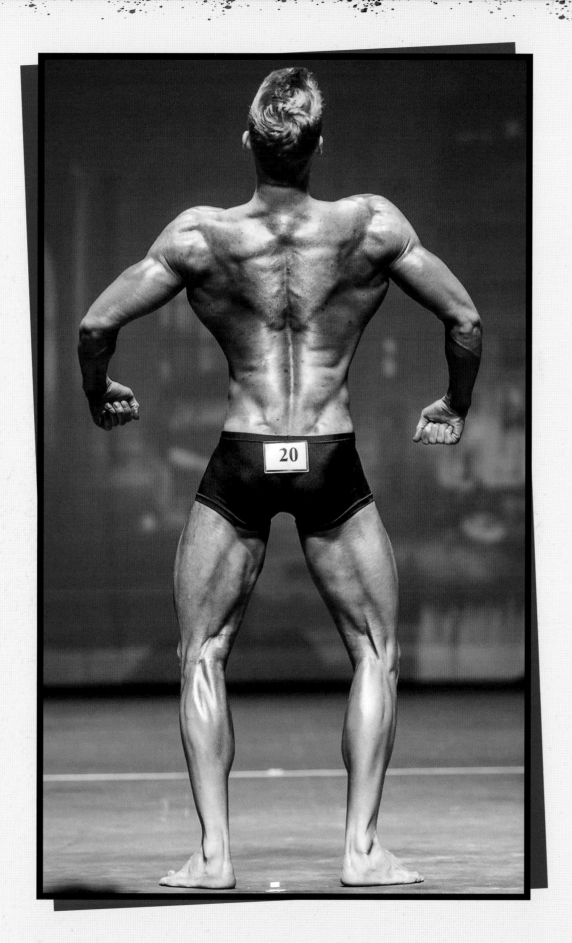

FRONT DOUBLE BICEPS

The front double biceps pose is often called first in the mandatory posing round. You can set your feet in one of two ways. You may either keep your legs stationary as they are in the front standing relaxed pose, or you may bring one leg forward to display the quad. Pull your ribcage up as you pull in your abdominal wall as far as you can. Raise your arms up to your sides, with your elbows just slightly in front of your torso. Flex your biceps with a slightly open fist and one arm extended a little higher than the other. Keep your chin up and your shoulders down.

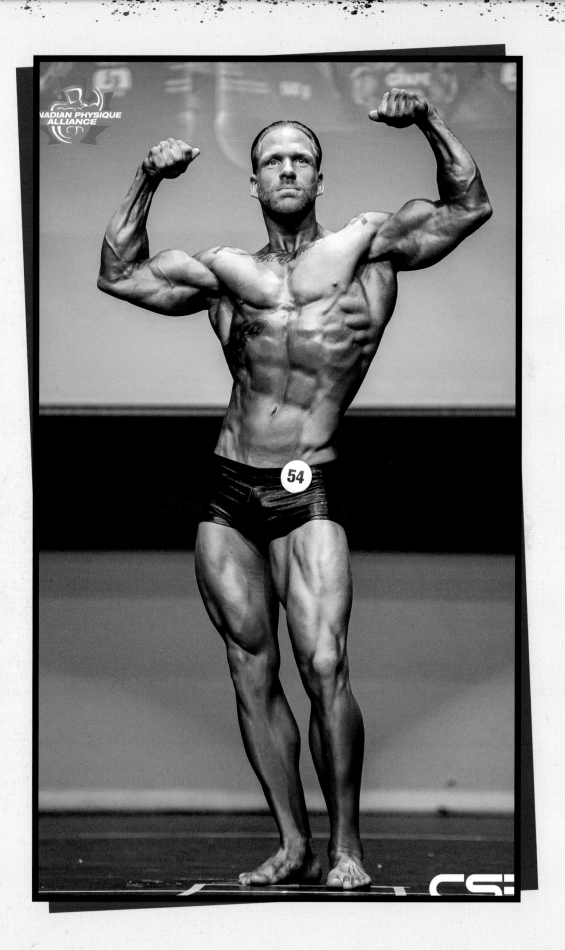

SIDE CHEST

After the front double biceps pose and front lat spread, the judges will ask you to quarter turn and face the side. The first pose usually called is the side chest pose. Spike the calf closest to the judges and squat down slightly. Your thigh should be at about a 35- to 55-degree angle to the floor. Take the knee furthest from the judges and push it slightly into your other leg. Flex the hamstring and glute closest to the judges. Place your ribcage in a neutral position while you flex your abs and intercostals and pull your abdomen inward as far as you can. Clasp your hands in front of you, and flex your pecs as you twist your torso ever so slightly toward the judges. Keep your shoulder down and your chin up.

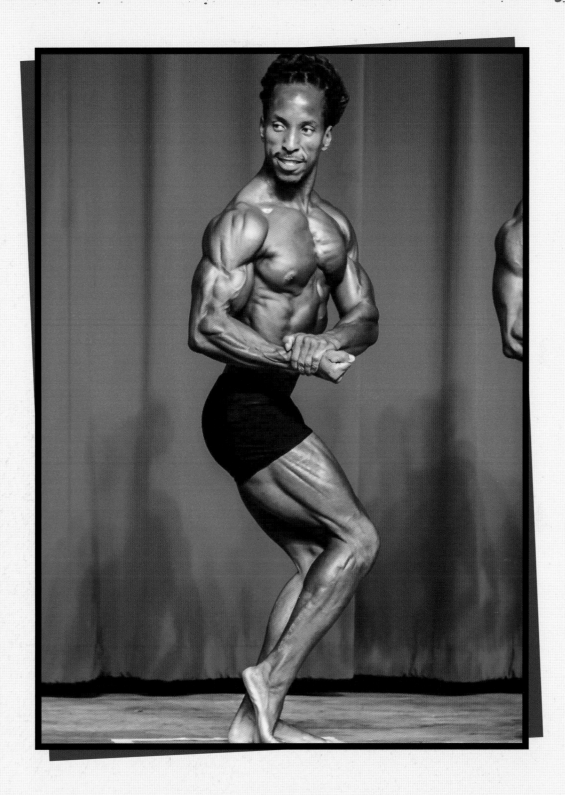

BACK (OR REAR) DOUBLE BICEPS

After you complete the side mandatory poses, the judges will have you quarter turn toward the back of the stage. Typically, they call out *rear double biceps pose*, sometimes called the *back double biceps pose*. Place one foot behind you and spike the calf. Sometimes the judges specify which calf you should spike. If they do not specify which foot to place behind, pick the one you feel most comfortable with. Place your foot behind your other foot approximately 10 to 15 inches (25-38 cm). Your knees should be turned outward slightly and bent just a little. Flex both hamstrings by digging your feet against the floor, as if you were trying to perform a leg curl. Flex and squeeze your glutes tightly. Bring your arms out to your sides and flex your biceps and the entire muscularity of your back. Keep your fists slightly open as you raise one arm a little higher than the other. You should not pinch your shoulder blades together. Instead, keep them open so that your back stays wide. Lean your torso back ever so slightly toward the judges.

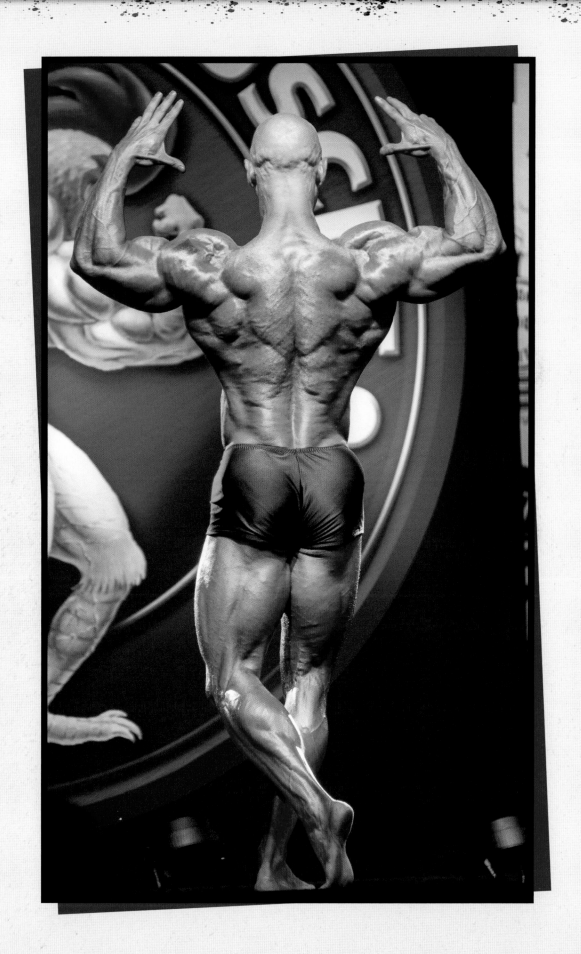

HANDS OVERHEAD ABDOMINAL
(OR AB AND THIGH)

After the back poses, the judges may have you perform the side chest and side triceps poses on the other side. Then they will bring you back around to the front for the hands overhead abdominal pose. This pose is also sometimes called the *ab and thigh pose*. Begin by placing one leg in front of the other and spiking the calf. Sometimes the judge may specify which leg they want to see. If they do not specify which leg to place forward, use the leg you are most comfortable with. Flex the quads in both legs, but make sure you prominently display the quads on the forward leg. Raise your hands and place them behind your head. Then flex your abs as hard as you can while you slightly crunch down to increase the contraction. Keep your pecs and arms flexed and your arms as close as possible to your head.

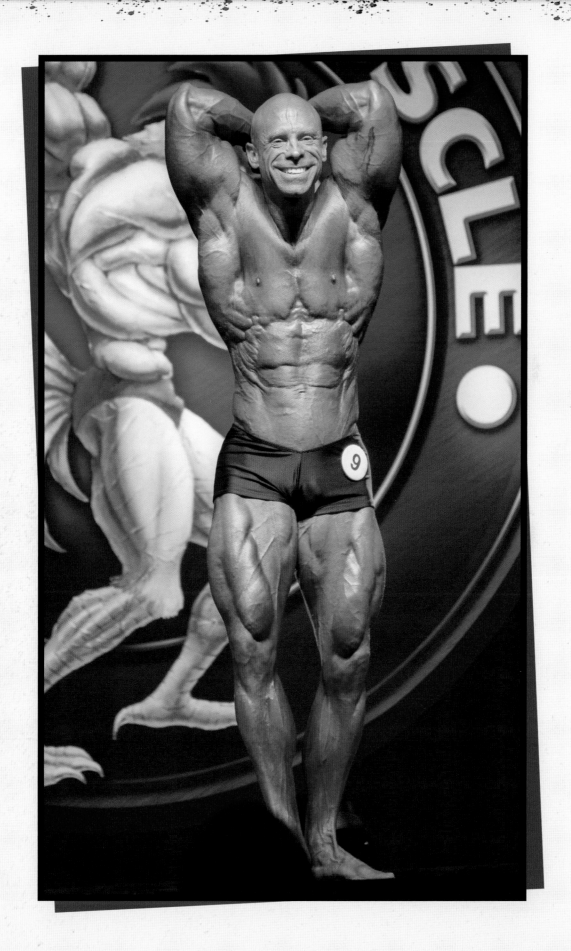

FAVORITE CLASSIC POSE

The classic physique division is different from the other divisions in that one of the mandatory poses is self-selected. Competitors are encouraged to be creative with this pose; however, we recommend choosing a pose that best showcases strengths in your physique. Three potential options appear here; however, there are many other poses you can hit as your favorite classic pose. Typically, the only pose that is not allowed as a favorite classic pose is a most muscular. Check with the sanction for your competition for clarification on what poses cannot be used as a favorite classic pose.

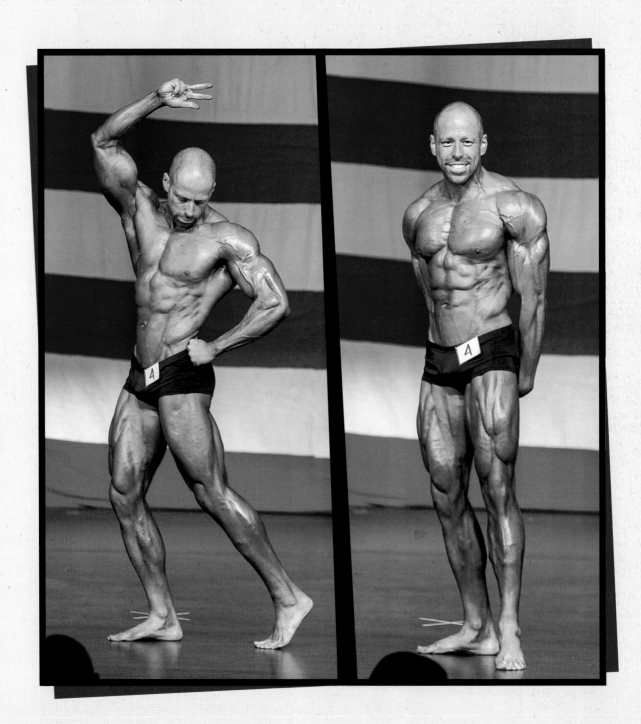

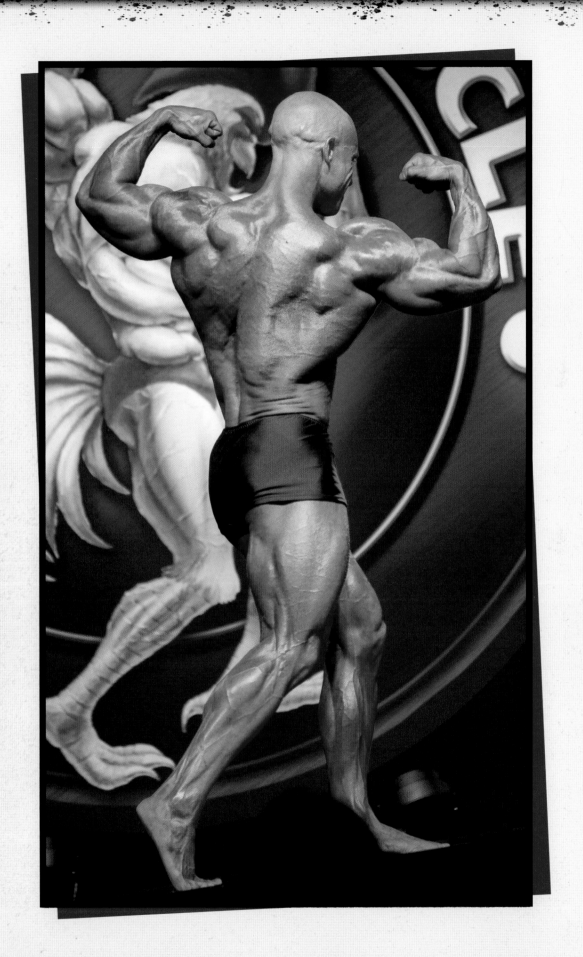

FRONT POSE

The first pose in men's physique is the front pose. This pose can be done a few ways. You should stand with your feet facing the judges and set about shoulder-width apart. Flex and pull in the abs very tightly because the abs are one of the primary areas of focus in men's physique. You should then slightly twist your hips so that you can give the illusion of a smaller waist. Do not twist too much, or the judges may ask you to face the front. Make sure to flare your lats. Your hands can then either be out to your sides, or you may have one hand on your hip. Keep your chin up and your shoulders down. Your smile should look genuine.

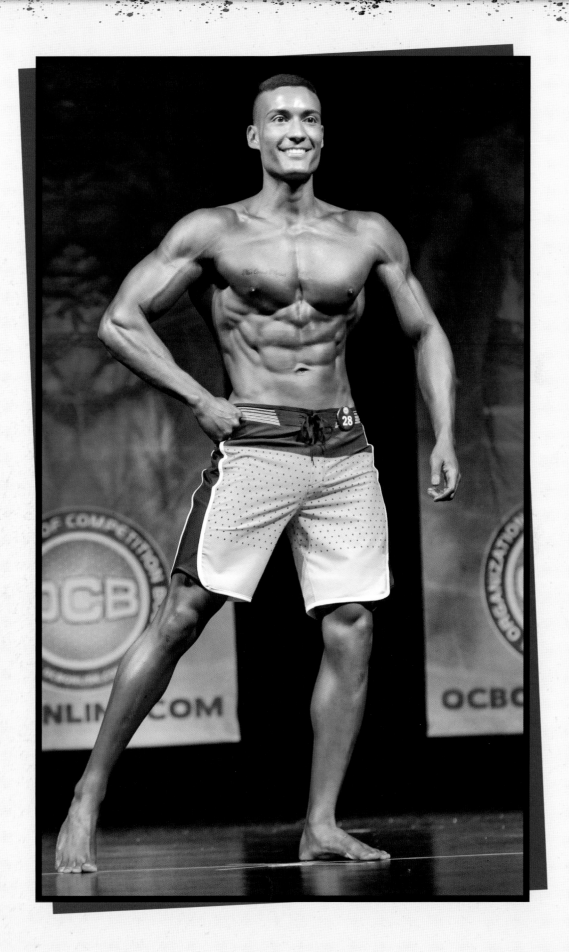

SIDE POSE

After you complete the front pose, the judge will ask you to quarter turn to the right. You then go into the side pose. With this pose, you should turn your feet to face the side of the stage and keep your hips squared toward the side of the stage. Then rotate your shoulders to face the judges while strongly flexing your abs and intercostals. You can either have both arms at your sides or one hand on your hip. Turn your head toward the judges and keep your chin up. Your smile should look genuine.

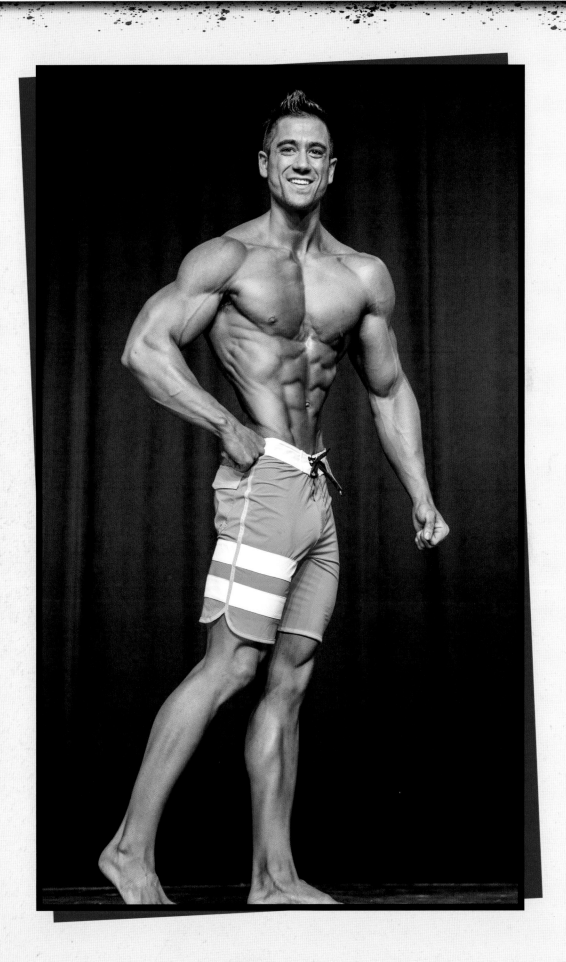

BACK POSE

After the side pose, you will be asked to quarter turn once again and face the back of the stage for the back pose. You should have your feet and hips facing toward the back of the stage. Lift your ribcage up as high as you can and flare your lats as you flex them. Your arms should be out toward your sides at about a 45-degree angle. You have the option to place one hand on your hip. Lean back very slightly and keep your head up.

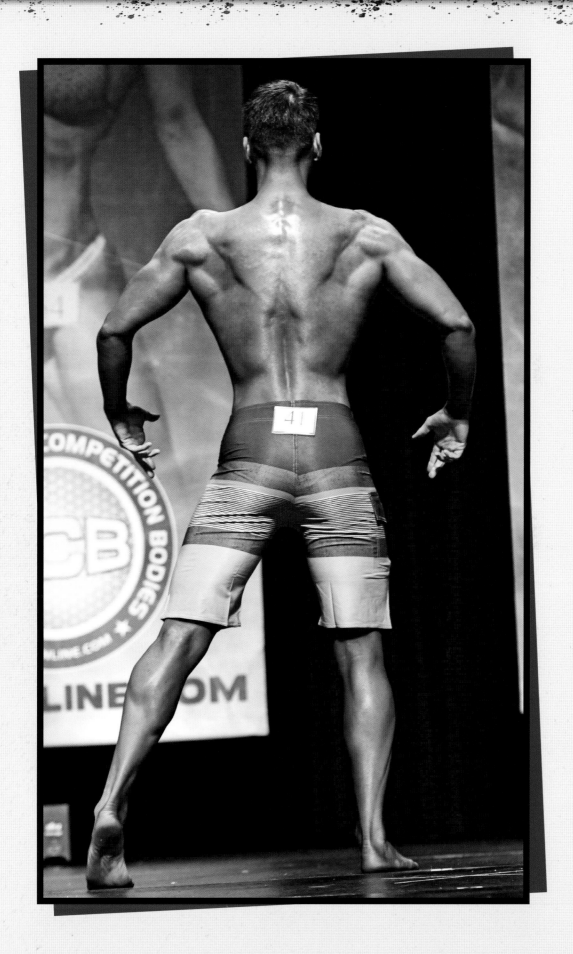

FRONT STANDING RELAXED

When you first walk out on stage with the other competitors, you will be lined up, and you should immediately execute the front standing relaxed pose. The judges will not call out this pose because you are expected to go directly into it.

To properly perform a front standing relaxed pose, face the judges. When executing any pose, run through a checklist of where your body parts should be from the ground up. As you face the judges, set your feet just a bit narrower than shoulder width, with your toes slightly turned outward to enhance quad sweep. Flex your quads, pushing your feet against the ground, almost as if you were trying to push your feet through the floor. Shift your hips back ever so slightly so they cause separation in your upper quads. Next, raise your ribcage as high as you can and pull your abdominal wall in as far as you can. Imagine trying to touch your navel to your spine. Flare your lats and keep your arms out at your sides at roughly a 45-degree angle, your hands open. Do not make a fist. Keep your shoulder girdle down, keep your chin up, and aim to have a relaxed facial expression in all poses.

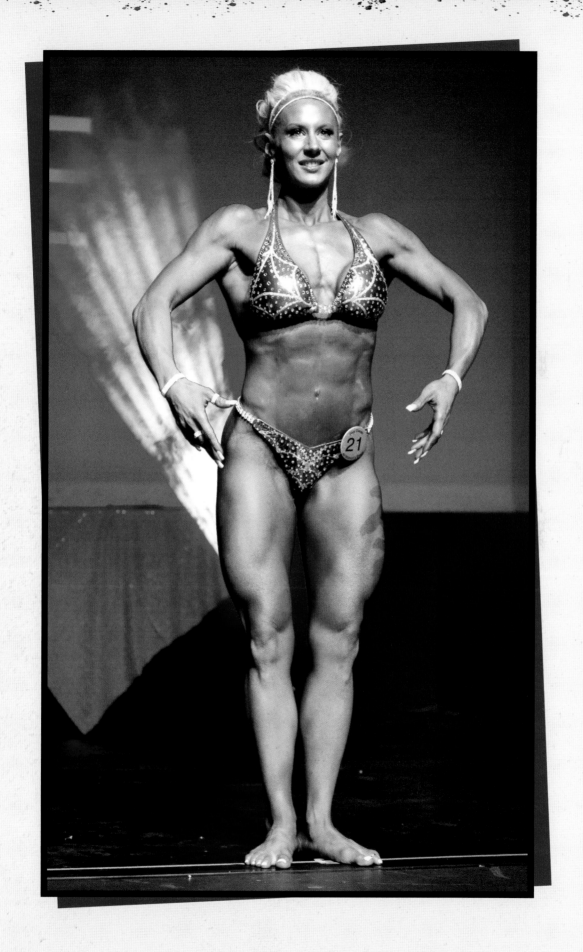

SIDE STANDING RELAXED

After the front standing relaxed pose, the judges will say, "Quarter turn." Always turn to the right. Then go directly into the side standing relaxed pose.

Start the side standing relaxed pose by facing the side of the stage. Your feet should be touching or almost touching, with the foot closest to the judges about one or two inches (2.5-5 cm) in front of the other foot. Slightly bend the knee closest to the judges. Keeping your rib cage down or in a neutral position, flex your abs and pull your abdominal wall in as far as you possibly can. Flex your pecs and turn your shoulders very slightly to open up to the judges. Use your back arm to slightly push into your back pectoral. Do not make a fist. Keep your chin up and your head facing to the side of the stage. Do not look at the judges in the side standing relaxed pose.

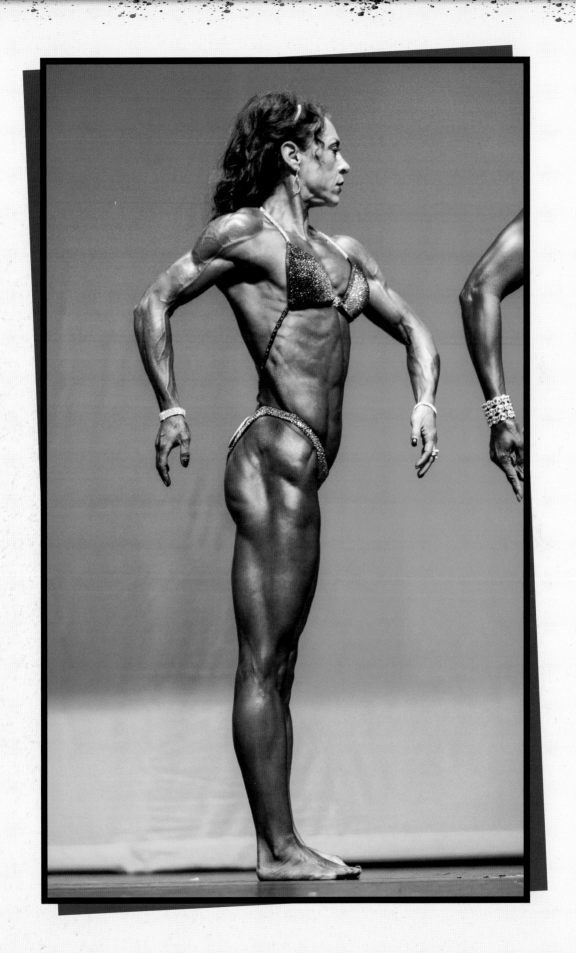

REAR STANDING RELAXED

After the side standing relaxed, the judges will say, "Quarter turn to the right." You should face the back of the stage with your back toward the judges and then go into the rear standing relaxed pose. Start with your feet just narrower than shoulder width. Turn your toes slightly out to the sides so that your outer quads will be visible from the back. Bend your knees a little and flex your hamstrings by imagining pressing your heels backward. You should then squeeze your glutes. Flare and flex your lats as you bring your arms to your sides at roughly a 45-degree angle and open your hands. Do not make a fist. Lean back ever so slightly and keep your head up.

After your rear standing relaxed, the judges will once again say, "Quarter turn." You will face the other side. At this point, perform your side standing relaxed pose while facing the other direction.

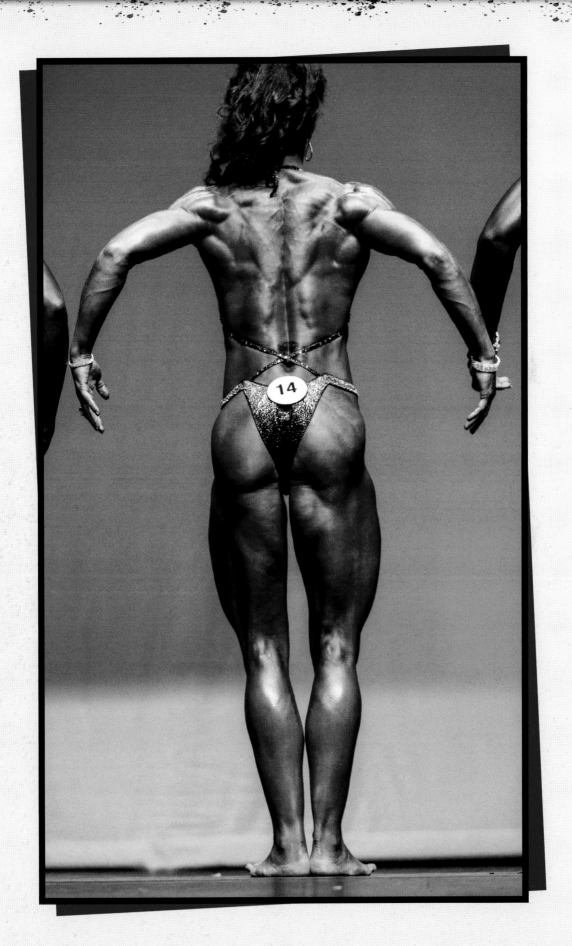

FRONT DOUBLE BICEPS

The front double biceps pose is often called first in the mandatory posing round. You can set your feet in one of two ways. You may either keep your legs stationary as they are in the front standing relaxed pose, or you may bring one leg forward to display the quad. Pull your ribcage up as you pull in your abdominal wall as far as you can. Raise your arms up to your sides with your elbows just slightly in front of your torso. Flex your biceps with a slightly open fist and one arm extended a little higher than the other. Keep your chin up and your shoulders down.

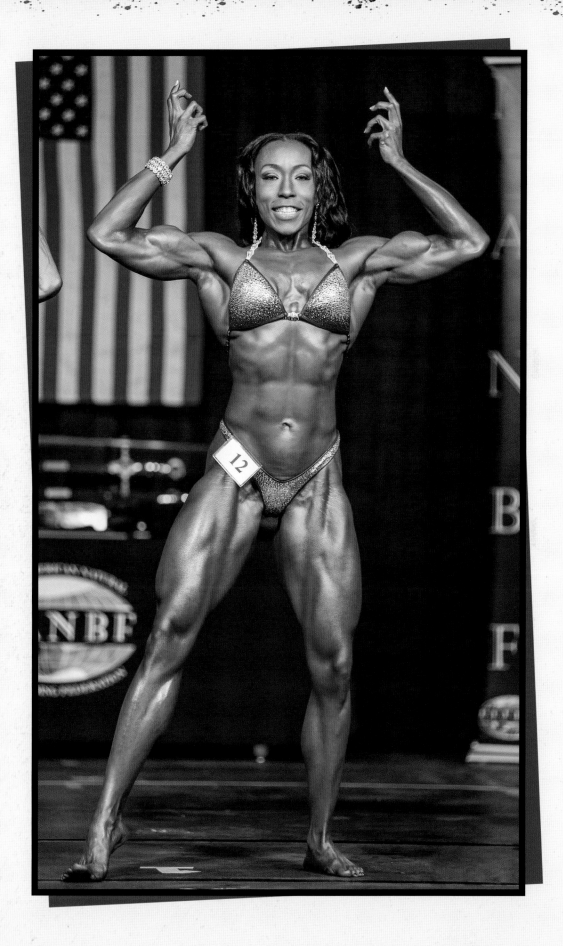

SIDE CHEST WITH LEG EXTENDED

After the front double biceps pose, the judges will ask you to quarter turn and face the side. The first pose usually called is the side chest pose. In this pose, fully extend the leg closest to the judges and flex the quads. Your thigh should be at about a 35- to 55-degree angle to the floor as you squat down just slightly. Place your ribcage in a neutral position while you flex your abs and intercostals and pull your abdomen inward as far as you can. Extend your hands in front of you, with your arms straight out and flex your pecs and triceps as you twist your torso ever so slightly toward the judges. Keep your shoulder down and your chin up.

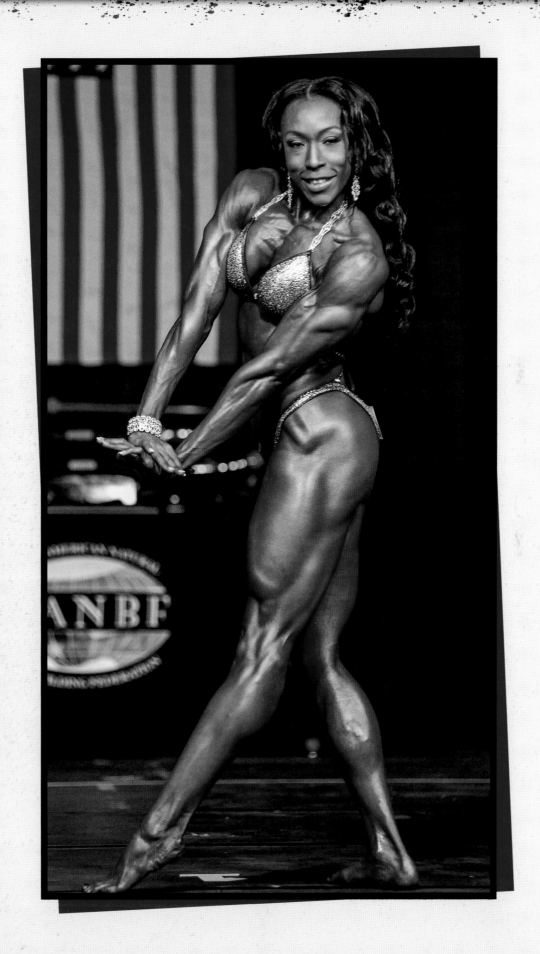

SIDE TRICEPS WITH LEG EXTENDED

The side triceps pose begins with your feet and legs set just as they are in the side chest pose, with one leg fully extended and quads flexed. However, instead of clasping your hands in front, you clasp them behind your back. You can do this by either locking your fingers together or using your back hand to grab the wrist of your front hand. Keep your torso in an upright position as you flex your abs and intercostals while pulling your abdominal wall in as far as you can. Open your body ever so slightly toward the judges but do not pull your arm behind you. Your goal should be to display the triceps prominently to the judges. Do not shrug your shoulders; this is a common mistake. Keep your chin up.

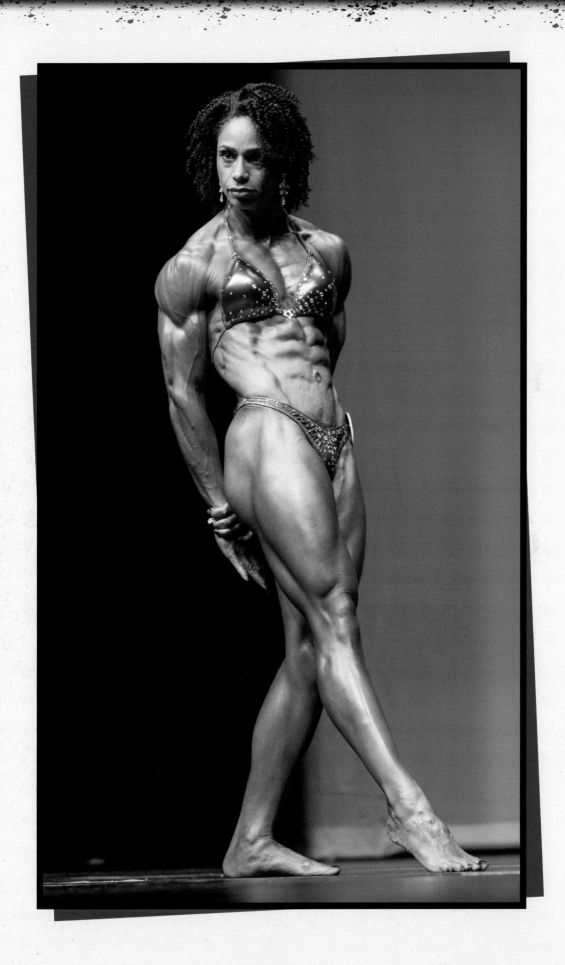

BACK (OR REAR) DOUBLE BICEPS

After you complete the side mandatory poses, the judges will have you quarter turn toward the back of the stage. Typically, they then call out *rear double biceps pose*, sometimes called the *back double biceps pose*. Place one foot behind you and spike the calf. Sometimes the judge specifies which calf you should spike. If he or she does not specify which foot to place behind, pick the one you feel most comfortable with. Place your foot behind your other foot approximately 10 to 15 inches (25-38 cm). Your knees should be turned outward slightly and bent just a little. Flex both hamstrings by digging your feet against the floor, as if you were trying to perform a leg curl. Flex and squeeze your glutes tightly. Bring your arms out to your sides and flex your biceps and the entire muscularity of your back. Keep your fists slightly open as you raise one arm a little higher than the other. You should not pinch your shoulder blades together. Instead, keep them open so that your back stays wide. Lean your torso back ever so slightly toward the judges.

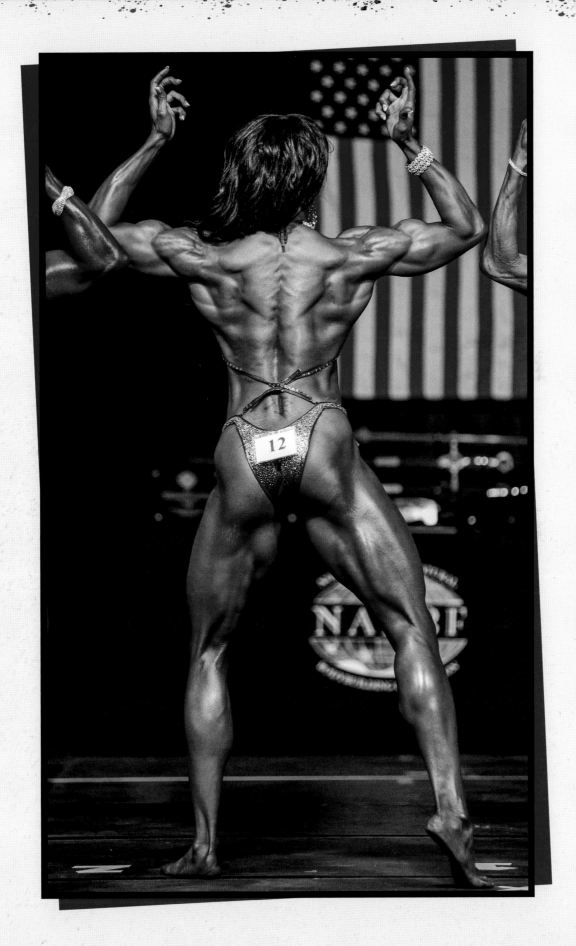

HANDS OVERHEAD ABDOMINAL (OR AB AND THIGH)

After the back poses, the judges may have you perform the side chest and side triceps poses on the other side. Then they bring you back around to the front for the hands overhead abdominal pose. This pose is also sometimes called the *ab and thigh pose*. Begin by placing one leg in front of the other and spiking the calf. Sometimes the judges specify which leg they want to see. If they do not specify which leg to place forward, use the leg you are most comfortable with. Flex the quads in both legs, but make sure you prominently display the quads on the forward leg. Raise your hands and place them behind your head. Then flex your abs as hard as you can while you slightly crunch down to increase the contraction. Keep your pecs and arms flexed as you perform this pose.

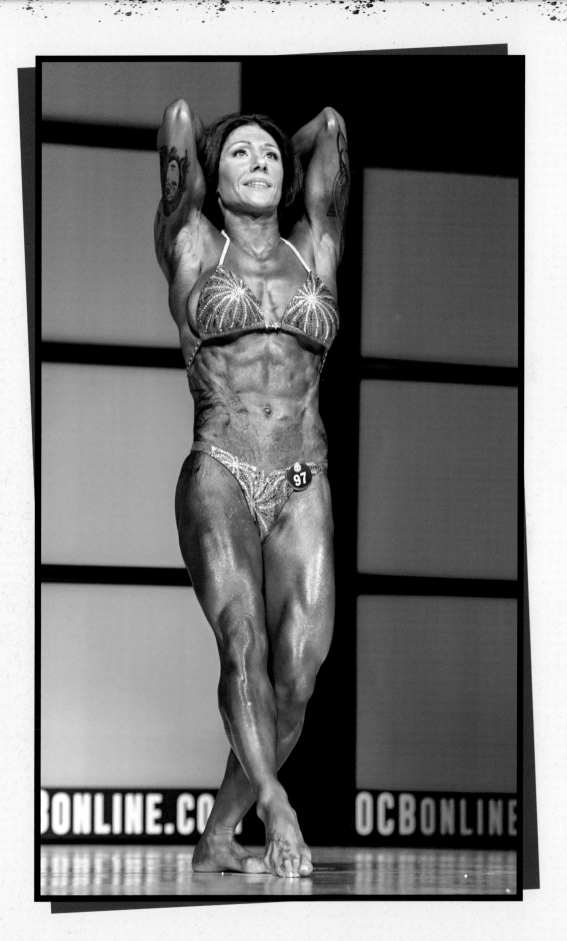

FRONT POSE

The first pose you do is the front pose. To start this pose, you should have your feet together. Your quads should be flexed, your hips slightly shifted back. Pull the ribcage up and pull in your abdomen as far as you can. The lats should be flared, with your arms out to your sides at about a 35- to 45-degree angle. The arms should be flexed but not rigid. Keep your shoulders down and your chin up. Your smile should look genuine.

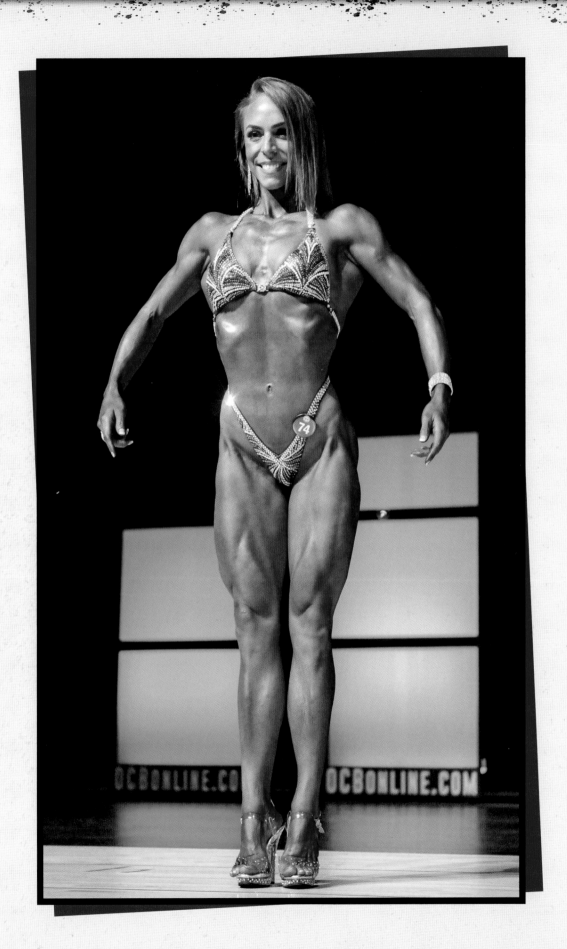

SIDE POSE

After the front pose, you will quarter turn to the right to face the side of the stage for the side pose. Keep your feet together and flex your quads, hamstrings, and glutes. Keep your ribcage up and your abs pulled in. Keep your arms flexed but not rigid. Open your torso very slightly toward the judges. Keep your chin up and shoulders down. Smile but do not turn your head toward the judges on the side pose.

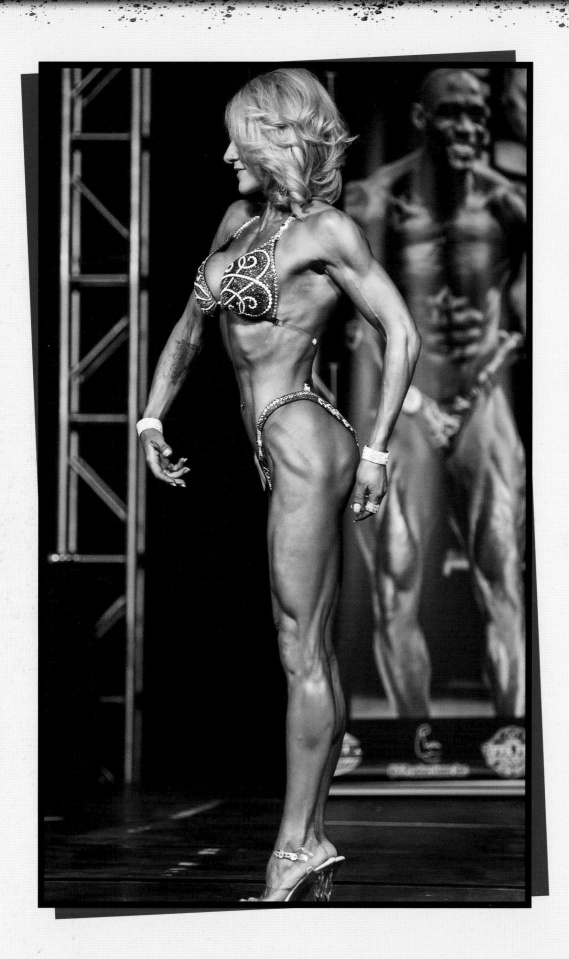

BACK POSE

The figure back pose should begin with your feet together, and your hair, if it is down, should be swept out of the way so the judges can see your whole back. Keep the hamstrings and glutes flexed, with your hips slightly shifted back. Shifting the hips causes the skin on the glutes to tighten, which is important. Pull the ribcage up while you flex and flare your lats. Keep your arms flexed but not rigid. Your shoulders should be down and your chin up.

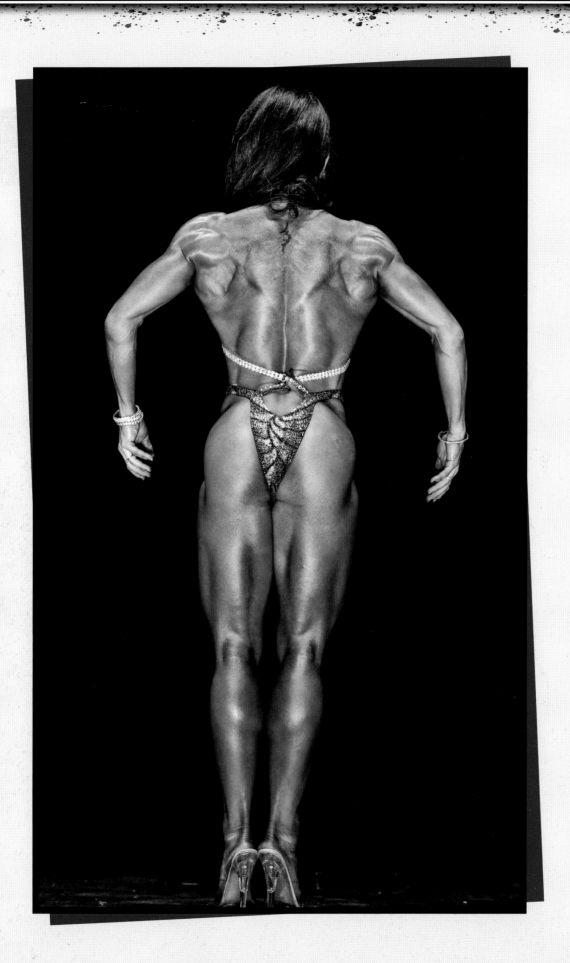

FRONT POSE

When executing the front pose in bikini, the goal is to minimize the width of your waist as much as possible while displaying the width of your shoulders. This is where the subtlety of bikini posing and individuality can be a key factor. Place your feet approximately shoulder-width apart. Shift your hips to one side. This maximizes the amount of curve displayed on your physique. Pull your abs in as far as possible and twist your hips away from the judges to show the smallest part of your waist. If possible, do not square your hips directly toward the judges. Lift your ribcage high as your shoulders face the judges. Your arms can either be out at the sides or one hand may be placed on the hip. Be sure to smile and display confidence.

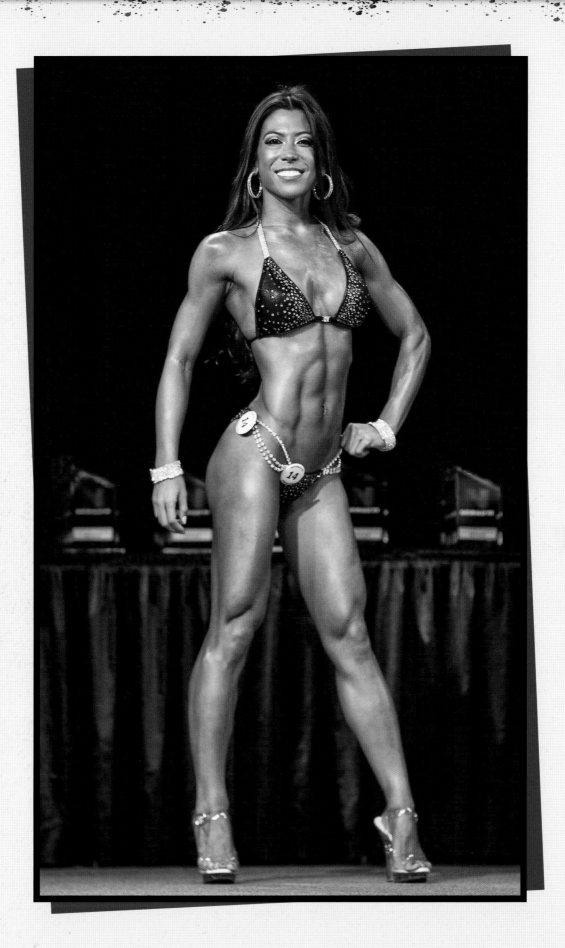

BACK POSE

The back pose for bikini is just as subtle as the front pose. When the judges ask you to half turn, you should transition smoothly to face the back of the stage. Once you are facing the back of the stage, your feet should be about shoulder-width apart or slightly wider. Your hair, if it is down, should be swept out of the way to display your back musculature. Shift your hips back to tighten your hamstrings and glutes, but do not bend over. Arch your back, with your chest and ribcage up. Slightly flex your back and arms while making it look natural and effortless.

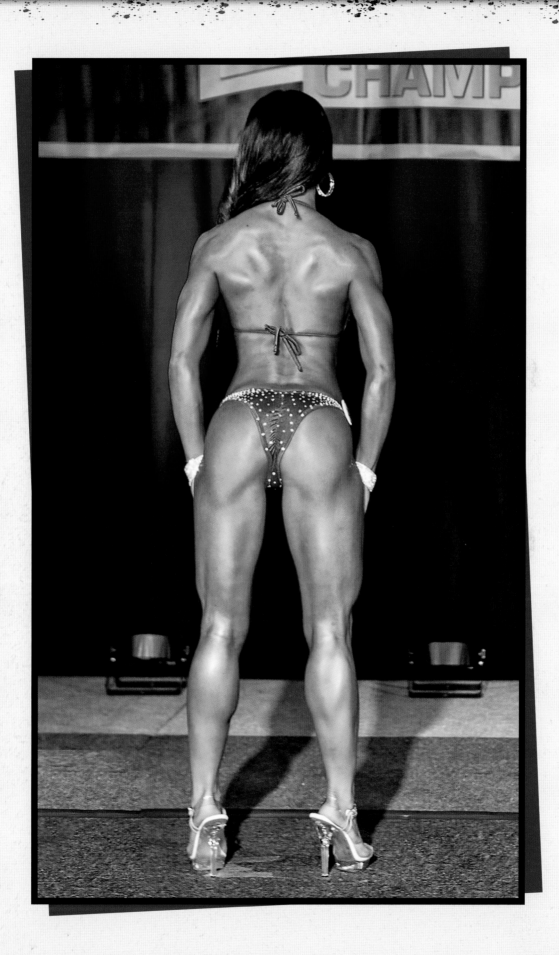

POSING ROUTINES AND T-WALKS

Every bodybuilding show will have a round for posing routines and T-walks. This round can vary depending on which sanction you compete in. In some sanctions, posing routines are mandatory, in some they are optional, and others only allow the top five to perform a routine. Check the rules of your sanctioning organization. In most sanctions, posing routines are not judged. They are purely for enjoyment. There are a few sanctions where the routines are judged and scored, so once again, check the rules of your sanctioning organization. You will not perform both a routine and a T-walk. Some divisions perform routines, and others do T-walks.

Posing Routines

Posing routines are performed in men's and women's bodybuilding, classic physique, and women's physique.

A typical posing routine is usually about 30 to 90 seconds long, depending on the sanction you are competing in. Often, you choose your own music and need to prepare a copy to bring with to the show. However, check with the show promoter because some shows play house music for everyone.

During your routine, you should present your body to your best ability by hitting poses that highlight your strengths and hide your weaknesses. For example, if you have a weak back, but your chest and quads are good, put more front poses into your routine and very few back poses, if any. Aim to execute the poses that you think are your best while staying away from your worst poses. Transitions between poses should be smooth and seem effortless. Have a plan for poses that can be easily executed and quickly transitioned into the next pose.

It is often better to perform a good but shorter routine that highlights your best areas rather than to have it go on too long and possibly expose your weak areas. You do not need to use all your allotted time. If you are allowed 60 seconds but only need 45 seconds to effectively perform your routine, you can wave to the audience and walk off the stage to end your routine.

T-Walks

T-walks are performed in figure, men's physique, and bikini. T-walks are different from posing routines, but both have the goal of presenting your body to your best ability by hitting poses that highlight your strengths and hide your weaknesses. Aim to execute the poses that you think are your best while staying away from your worst poses.

The name *T-walk* comes from the points in which you walk across the stage. With posing routines, you are allowed to use the entire stage; however, with T-walks, you have specific marks on the stage where you must stop and execute a pose. Each show will have a slightly different set of rules for how and where you enter onto the stage. Therefore, be flexible.

There is usually a point in the back center of the stage where the first pose will be executed. You do not have to perform any specific pose; instead, you can choose the poses that highlight your physique at each mandated spot. After your first pose, you will usually either be asked to walk toward the front center of the stage or break off to the left or right to the next spot. As stated earlier, the exact order in which you will be asked to walk is up to the show promoter or the sanction. However, the points you hit will be back center, front center, left of stage, and right of stage. You should have one or two poses prepared for each spot. Most T-walks are allotted 60 to 90 seconds. Make sure you know your time and use it accordingly.

EFFECTIVE PRACTICE POSING

When preparing for a bodybuilding show, practicing your posing is a crucial part of setting yourself up for success. All too often, people devote hours and hours to practicing for a show, but they are not actually practicing *effectively*. You should not only work hard at your posing and put in the time but also know precisely what you need to accomplish with all that effort and time invested. This is where most competitors go wrong. Let us look at the two major components to proper posing practice and how to execute them.

Practicing Posing Technique

Often, newer competitors spend hours practicing posing and making sure they can hold a pose for lengthy periods of time; however, the pose they are holding is poorly executed and will cost them points onstage. In this case, all time and effort have been wasted.

Before you focus on being able to hold poses, practice how to effectively perform the poses. Although we gave you a rundown of how to execute the poses in the previous sections, that is only a basic description of how to pose. Posing is a lot like trying on clothes: While a shirt or a pair of pants may be tailored the same way, the subtleties of how it looks on different bodies can either make it a great fit or a terrible fit.

To fine-tune your posing, you must practice. Start with the base example of the poses we listed previously, and then try slight variations to see how they look. This is simply a process of trial and error. Little things like seeing what happens if you raise your hands slightly higher or lower, place your elbows slightly forward or backward, or turn your feet inward or outward a bit more can all have a profound effect from person to person. The goal of practicing posing technique is to find the precise way that each pose looks best for you. Experimentation is the key here.

We recommend beginning practicing posing technique at least from the first day of your contest prep or, even better, starting in the off-season. Spend at least 10 to 15 minutes each day trying out various techniques. In this stage of posing practice, you do not need to worry about holding your poses. Instead, simply practice various hand, foot, and elbow placements, or even try various ways of flexing different body parts. Over time, you will find what looks best for you.

> ## FAQ: Should I practice the poses while wearing my posing suit?
>
> Yes, you should practice posing in your suit. Being on stage feels uncomfortable for many. You should make everything as close to how it will be on show day as possible so that you are completely comfortable when you get out there.

Practicing Posing Conditioning

Over the course of your entire prep and possibly your off-season, work on your posing technique. However, starting eight weeks out, your focus should switch from posing technique to posing conditioning. This is where you condition yourself to be able to hold your poses onstage without tiring. It is not often talked about, but this is typically a grueling part of contest prep. Posing can be exhausting and painful. If you fail to practice, you will not be able to flex and hold your poses effectively onstage without tiring. It is common to see a competitor come onstage and look amazing. However, as the comparison rounds drag on, you can see him or her begin to fade because he or she is tiring and is not as sharp or perhaps is unable to continue flexing since exhaustion is setting in. Many times, you also see shaking as a result. To avoid this, you must practice.

The following are our recommendations for how to structure your posing conditioning practice.

The Setup

Since you have already been practicing your posing technique, you should easily be able to execute each pose. At this stage of your prep, begin practicing posing without looking at a mirror. There will be no mirror onstage, so you need to start learning how to pose without looking at yourself. We recommend setting up a video camera or using your smartphone to record your sessions. This way, you can pose without looking at yourself, but you can then watch the session later to see what mistakes you may have made.

The Execution

The important part of posing conditioning practice is to pose nonstop for a specified period. We recommend that you simply simulate show day. This means to practice running through the standing relaxed and mandatory comparison poses because the judge will call them on show day. Each time you hit a pose and then relax, you should return to your standing relaxed pose. You need to push yourself to keep posing hard, just as you will on show day. Continue running through all the poses repeatedly until your time is up.

The Timing

To start your posing practice, we recommend that at eight weeks out, you begin by posing as described above for nine minutes continuously every day. This should be difficult to start but achievable. From that point, you should aim to add one and a half minutes to your time every fourth day. This means that after four days, you start posing for 10-1/2 minutes each day; by the eighth day, you begin posing for 12 minutes each day; and beginning on the twelfth day, you will pose for 13-1/2 minutes each; and so on. If you continue in this fashion, by show day, you should be able to hold your poses for 30 minutes straight without stopping at all. If you pushed yourself hard during your posing practice, you will be more than ready to handle whatever the judges throw at you on show day.

FAQ: Should I pose in a sauna?

People pose in a sauna to lose water weight. If this is the intention, we do not recommend it. However, posing in a sauna or possibly in a bathroom with a hot shower running has the advantage of helping you practice in heat. The lights on stage are typically hot, and you will be sweaty. It can be a new sensation for a lot of competitors who are used to being cold while posing. Just make sure you shorten your posing duration slightly if you do pose in a sauna and stay well hydrated.

Take-Home Points

▶ Proper posing can make or break your placing onstage. Therefore, understand what the judges are looking for in each pose within your division.

▶ In most competitions, you need to also prepare a posing routine or T-walk. Competitors in men and women's bodybuilding, classic physique, and women's physique do posing routines, but competitors in men's physique, figure, and bikini do T-walks. The details of posing routines and T-walks may differ from sanction to sanction, so consult the show details for more information.

▶ Posing practice is critical to your success onstage. Begin posing technique practice either in the off-season or at the start of contest prep to ensure that you are performing each pose in a way that best suits your physique. At eight weeks out, begin working on practicing posing conditioning, where you then hold your poses for increasing periods of time. This ensures you can handle whatever the judges throw at you on show day.

The Finishing Touches and Final Preparation

There is a difference between competing and being a competitor. True competitors leave no stone unturned. They step on stage looking polished and leaving no doubt that they are truly ready. This all comes down to the small details. During contest prep, your focus should be on being consistent with your nutrition and training and adjusting as necessary to keep progressing toward looking your best on show day. However, other considerations during contest prep should be addressed before the day of the contest so show day goes as smoothly as possible. This chapter covers these less-discussed details of contest prep.

POSING PRACTICE

As discussed in the previous chapter, you should begin to practice your posing technique in the off-season or, at least, at the start of contest prep to be sure you are performing poses in a way that best shows your physique. Once you are comfortable with your posing technique, practice holding poses for a longer time. This will ensure that you are ready for anything thrown your way on show day.

POSING MUSIC

You will also need to begin putting together a posing routine prior to your competition. What is expected and allowed in a posing routine differs between divisions and sanctions, so it is vital to find out the details for your specific competition. In addition, the importance of a posing routine differs from sanction to sanction. Some sanctions judge the posing routine (so you will need to put more emphasis on practicing your routine), while others do not judge posing routines. Moreover, some shows may not have you do a routine at all, or it may only be optional.

If you need to bring your own music, be sure that you put together your music—well in advance of show day—cut to where you plan on starting your routine. Most shows will ask you to either supply your music as a CD or MP3. However, some shows may only have house music played for all competitors during their routine. When in doubt, check with the sanction or show you plan to compete in for more information.

Pick music that you enjoy and that does not contain inappropriate language. Base the type of music you use on the type of routine you plan to perform and your physique. For example, if you are a mass monster hitting most muscular variants left and right, something like hard rock is going to be a good choice. However, if you have a more aesthetic physique and plan to hit a number of classic and nonmandatory poses, a more instrumental music selection may be best. However, there is no right or wrong choice here, and most of the time the routine is not judged so you can feel free to make it your own.

POSING SUIT

Competitors in each division wear a different type of posing suit. For example, a bikini competitor has a different posing suit than a figure competitor does, and a men's physique competitor has a different posing suit than a male bodybuilder does. The types of posing suits required or even allowed in a division may differ between sanctions. Consult the information provided by your sanction before ordering your suit.

If you plan to purchase a posing suit, order it at least 12 weeks before your competition. This gives the suit manufacturer time to receive your measurements, make your suit, and send it to you. You then have enough time to try on your suit and send back for alterations, if necessary.

Posing suits can be expensive, especially for female competitors. To cut costs, some competitors with fashion sense and sewing skills may make their own suits. There are also suit rental services available for those looking for another cost-effective solution.

SHOES

Women in bikini and figure need to purchase clear heels. Generally, four- or five-inch (10-13 cm) heels are recommended because they help create the illusion of elongated legs more so than shorter heels. Many women may not be comfortable wearing such a high heel, so it may be helpful to wear heels more frequently during daily life to increase comfort. Ultimately, a competitor needs to be comfortable enough in heels so that it does not look like she is struggling as she walks around onstage because this can negatively affect placing.

JEWELRY

Competitors in bikini and figure should purchase jewelry that sparkles under the stage lights. Jewelry worn onstage can be described as "over the top" or "costume jewelry." However, competitors can find cheap, shiny jewelry without having to spend much money. Those with questions about stage jewelry should consult the information provided by the sanction for their class, pictures and video from previous competitions within the sanction they plan to compete, or both.

HAIR REMOVAL

Removal of body hair is necessary to see muscle detail under stage lighting. Even fine, light-colored hair can affect a competitor's appearance onstage and should be removed before competition. There are several different hair removal methods available, such as shaving, waxing, and laser removal, among others.

Those who plan to shave should avoid doing the first shave immediately before the show. This is especially true for males with a lot of hair to remove. The initial shave often results in razor burn or cuts, especially for those who are inexperienced; therefore, it may be advisable to begin shaving a couple of weeks before the competition to avoid razor burn and cuts on show day.

TANNING

The ideal type of tan depends on your skin complexion, preference, and the division you will compete in. In general, the more extreme the look required for your division, the darker your tan needs to be because a dark tan helps show more detail under the bright stage lights. Bodybuilders need to be extremely dark while those competing in bikini should aim for a more natural look under stage lights. However, even a natural look onstage needs to be significantly darker than normal skin pigmentation for most competitors. Competitors in classes such as figure or men's physique should strive to find a middle ground.

Tanning Products

There are number of different options for self-tanning products, and most competitions provide tanning services for a fee. Most self-tanning products fall into two categories.

Oil-Based Products

The most common oil-based tanning product is Dream Tan. This product does not absorb into the skin or dry well, which makes it a poor choice for the bikini and men's physique divisions. However, it does provide a very dark color and a shine due to the oil in the product. Dream Tan is not allowed at all competitions. Make sure you check the rules for your show to ensure it is allowed.

Stain-Based Products

Unlike oil-based tanning products, stain-based products absorb into the skin and dry well. They stick on the skin and leave the skin darker for a few days after the competition. The most common stain-based products are Pro Tan, Jan Tana, and Dark As. Pro Tan and Jan Tana tend to give a lighter, more natural color under stage lights (keep in mind this will still be very dark when not under stage lighting). Dark As results in a much darker color, like oil-based products.

FAQ: Do all competitions allow the same type of tan?

Competitions may differ in the type of tanning product allowed. Some sanctions or competitions may not allow an oil-based tan. Consult information regarding your specific competition for more information on the type of tanning products allowed.

Other Considerations

Those using stain-based tanning products need oil to put over the tan before going onstage. Most stain-based products have an oil product recommended to use with the tanning product. Competitors using Dream Tan do not need to use oil because of the oil already in the product. (In fact, baby wipes are a great way to remove Dream Tan after a competition.)

Before using a particular self-tanning product you're not used to, do a practice run ahead of time so that you know you will be able to achieve your desired look when it counts.

FAQ: Do I need to get a base tan in a tanning bed before my competition?

For most tanning products, a base tan in a tanning bed is not necessary before competition. However, we would recommend following the guidelines provided by your tanning product of choice.

MAKEUP AND HAIR

Female competitors apply the tan up to the neck; the face is covered with makeup. This is likely significantly darker than what is worn in daily life to match the tan. In addition, a figure or bikini competitor's hair needs to be done in a way that makes it appear feminine (e.g., worn down). Many contests now provide services (for a fee) for makeup and hair that can remove the stress of doing them yourself on show day. However, these services book quickly, and appointments may fall behind on show day. If you are going to use these services, be on time for your appointments so that you are not the reason things fall behind.

For those doing their own makeup, look for what you will use ahead of time. Place some of your tanning product on your arm or leg before shopping for makeup. You should attempt to match the tan color as best as possible and err on the side of your makeup being slightly lighter than your tanning product but not drastically lighter to avoid having a white face and tan body onstage. Many competitors also purchase fake lashes and brightly colored lipstick. Ultimately, the overall look of your makeup for the stage needs to be much more drastic than daily life.

Competitors doing their own hair and makeup are also encouraged to practice ahead of time to be sure things go smoothly on show day. Ideas and makeup tips can often be found in online videos and tutorials.

Men may also need to determine their show-day hair products, depending on their hairstyles. Hair can be styled in the same way it is worn every day. Those with facial hair should be sure that it is nicely groomed.

OTHER LOGISTICAL DETAILS

When you are preparing for a show, failing to attend to the details that need your attention can, in the least, result in an inconvenience come show day, or, at the worst, result in you preparing for a show but not being allowed to compete. Just as you carefully prep your food and your training, be sure to handle other logistical details.

Contest Entry Form

Contest entry forms need to be mailed in before your competition. There are deadlines for regular entry and late entry (which is typically more expensive). Competitors choose which divisions and classes they enter on the form. Most competitions allow competitors to compete in more than one class as long as they are eligible and pay a crossover fee.

FAQ: When should I register for a show?

The deadline for show registration is around one or two weeks before a competition. We recommend consulting with the show promoter to be sure you meet the deadline. Since the deadline is typically close to a competition, a competitor can use this to his or her advantage. We recommend first-time competitors—or those who have not been stage-lean before—have multiple possible target shows (if possible). That way a competitor can select which show or shows he or she will compete in closer to the show date to be stage-lean by the competition time. We realize this may not be possible for all competitors due to schedules, location of competitions, and budget, but we still recommend not registering for a competition until you are sure you will be ready for it.

Sanction Card

Competitors also need to buy a sanction card and, if the contest is drug-tested, set up a time for their drug test (testing typically occurs on the day before the competition). A sanction card can usually be purchased at show check-in, and drug-testing times may not be set until closer to the show date. As a result, these tasks can be done after you register for the contest. Consult the promoter of your show for more information.

Travel and Hotel Arrangements

Unless you are one of the lucky few who can compete in your hometown, you will arrange for travel before your show. Most competitions have a host hotel that provides rooms at a discounted rate. However, do not feel you need to stay at the host hotel if you find a better option nearby. Before booking a hotel, make sure that your room has a refrigerator and microwave so that you can stay on track with your food plan in the last hours leading up to your show.

For most Saturday competitions, you should plan on arriving on Friday; however, if you are driving or flying long distances, it may be a good idea to arrive on Thursday. This gives any changes in water balance due to prolonged sitting time to regulate back to normal before you step onstage to ensure you are looking your best. In addition, arriving early can reduce stress and give you additional time to tie up any loose ends before show day.

Take-Home Point

▶ Many competitors focus on nutrition, training, cardio, and posing practice. However, there are several smaller details to address before show day. These include choosing music; scheduling drug testing and purchasing a sanction card; purchasing posing suits, shoes, and jewelry; getting a plan in place for tan, hair, and makeup on show day; and taking care of travel arrangements.

Peak Week Explained

It is Friday night, and you have a bodybuilding contest tomorrow. You have put in weeks and months of brutal hard work. However, rather than feeling the pride and excitement you should, your mind is consumed with one thought: "Dear God, please let this work!"

The next morning, you wake up and eagerly head over to the mirror. Your heart drops; it is not a pretty sight. The once-glorious striations on display only a week ago are now gone. The full and hard muscle bellies are replaced with a soft, smooth, and saggy look. Everything just looks off.

You hope that things look better once you get backstage and get a pump. "That will surely fix the problem!" you tell yourself. Even though you are trying to convince yourself all you need is to get a pump, you cannot help but run to a mirror every 10 minutes and check your conditioning, hoping something changes. It does not.

As stage time approaches, you head backstage, nervously strip down to your posing trunks, and begin pumping. As you pump feverishly and desperately, you begin to realize that absolutely nothing is happening. No matter how hard you try, you cannot get a pump.

With nothing else to do, you line up with the other competitors and take the stage. You are quickly moved to the end of the stage, where you remain until the end of prejudging.

As you head back to your hotel feeling defeated, your mind swirls with thoughts of what could have gone so wrong. Was your sodium off? Was it too many carbs or too few? Was it the water? You feel totally clueless about what you could have done differently.

This scenario is played out repeatedly, week after week, year in and year out. Bodybuilders often completely sabotage themselves in the final week. Even if things do not go terribly wrong, many competitors still notice they do not look as good on show day as they did a week before. Even if it is only a small difference, it is never a good feeling standing on stage knowing you could be better.

PEAK WEEK

Bodybuilders and other physique athletes can hardly be faulted for confusion and missteps regarding peak week. Most information that bodybuilders have about peak week comes from so-called bodybuilding gurus, secondhand advice from other competitors, and gym myths. Much of this is nothing more than pseudoscience or outright nonsense.

The lack of quality information also arises because there is no peer-reviewed research about peaking for a bodybuilding show. There are a couple of reasons for not having real research on the subject. First, peaking for a bodybuilding show is a niche subject for a very niche market. Finding funding for a study like this would be difficult.

Second, even if funding were available, determining what constitutes an optimal peak would be tough to quantify. It might be possible to conduct effective peaking research by stacking multiple measurements together, such as limb girth changes, BIA to measure total body water, DEXA, and possibly ultrasound (or, even better, a CT scan or MRI). If you combined these, you should be able to tell the difference in girth size, changes in body water, and, hopefully, where the water is being stored. Unfortunately, this brings us back to the issue of cost in executing so many different tests.

With this chapter, we will lift the veil of mystery surrounding peak week. We need to delve into the science behind the variables at play during peak week. We can use plenty of research and information about how the human body functions to extrapolate about how to properly peak.

In addition to examining the human body's function and processes, we offer insight from our years of experience. To date, we have coached hundreds of competitive physique athletes to the stage, including some of the top drug-free bodybuilders in the world. The things we have learned from these real-world experiences have been invaluable, and we look forward to sharing our findings.

PREREQUISITES FOR EFFECTIVE PEAKING

Peaking cannot simply be done at random. It cannot transform someone in only a week's time. Remember that it is called *peak week*, not *magic week*. It will not work miracles. An effective peak only enhances what you already have. There are three primary prerequisites for effective peaking. Before you even think about the possibility of peaking, you must meet these requirements.

Prerequisite 1: You Must Be Lean

This cannot be overemphasized and should be considered the absolute highest priority. Before you can peak effectively for a bodybuilding show, you must be lean, ripped, shredded, peeled, or any number of adjectives you use to describe someone who is lacking body fat.

We estimate that 90 to 95 percent of competitors are not lean enough going into peak week. Many competitors are quick to say, "Once I lose this water weight during peak week, I'll look great. " That statement is just dripping with wishful thinking. It is almost never water weight that needs to be lost; it is fat. If you see a pocket of fat anywhere on your body, then you need more diet time, plain and simple.

Prerequisite 2: Know Your Baseline Macronutrient Intake

Many competitors who follow meal plans go into a show knowing the type and quantity of foods they consume. For example, they may know that they eat eight ounces (227 g) of chicken and one cup (about 200 g) of cooked rice for a meal, but they do not actually know how much protein, carbs, and fat they are consuming daily. This is a problem because if you do not know your current intake, you will not be able to effectively cause change. Peaking is like reading a map. To get where you want to go, you need to know where you are right now.

Prerequisite 3: Know Your Approximate Daily Water and Sodium Intake

For the same reasons you must know your macronutrient intake, you must know your approximate daily intake of water and sodium. (Although you should know your *precise* intake for your macronutrient intake, you need a close approximation for water and sodium.) For the sake of precision, we suggest closely tracking water and sodium about two or three weeks before peak week. It is also a good idea to make sure your daily intake does not drastically fluctuate from day to day.

These three prerequisites are listed in order of importance. Being lean is the highest priority. If you are not lean enough, attempting to peak will be futile, and you will be better off simply picking a later show date to give yourself more time to get leaner.

TERMINOLOGY AND DEFINITIONS

Before discussing the specifics of various peaking plans, understand the terminology associated with peak week. We realize that terminology may not seem terribly important when trying to be your best on show day, but it is more integral than most people realize. For example, compare this to the medical field. If a nurse tells the doctor that a patient is dead when she really means that he is in a coma, the doctor will react differently based on that word. A medical professional must know the difference between death and a coma and accurately identify the state. Likewise, a bodybuilder needs to be able to know the difference between *flat* and *spilled* and be able to identify those states. Effective peaking requires a constant analysis of one's body state. If you cannot properly identify the state your body is in, it is impossible to make the correct adjustments.

A lot of terms have been used when talking about the process of peaking, but as far as we know, there is no complete list. The following are the common essential peaking terms and what they mean:

- ► *Flat:* Muscles are not round or full because the muscle tissue is not pushing tightly against the skin.
- ► *Full:* Muscles have a rounded appearance and are typically pushing out tightly against the skin.
- ► *Spilled (or spilled over):* Excess subcutaneous water is present under the skin. This blurs definition and reduces visible striations and separation between muscles. This is typically accompanied by a full look but not always.
- ► *Tight:* Skin is pulled tightly against muscle tissue with no signs of spilling or excessive subcutaneous water.
- ► *Vascular:* The visible protrusion of superficial veins and arteries.
- ► *Lean (or ripped or shredded):* The absence of visible subcutaneous body fat.
- ► *Holding water:* This is a common term in bodybuilding, but it is not clear because the body is made largely of water. We are always holding water. The important thing is *where* the water is being held. The term is typically given to someone who does not look good. In our experience, it is usually used as a catch-all for several different things that have gone wrong with a peak.

PEAK WEEK OBJECTIVES

You may find it a bit silly to have an entire section devoted to objectives. We can practically hear people thinking, "I only have one objective, bro, and that is to be huge and shredded." While this is an admirable goal, we need to get more specific with how this is actually accomplished to make it happen. When you break down each objective individually, a clearer picture of what is needed begins to take shape.

Our objectives for an effective peak week can be split into two different categories: primary and secondary. **Primary objectives** have the largest impact on whether our peak week will be a success or a failure. Therefore, they are of primary importance. **Secondary objectives** still have an impact on our physique but not to the degree of our primary objectives.

Primary Objective 1: Maximize Muscle Size and Fullness
You maximize muscle size and fullness through three mechanisms: optimizing glycogen storage, keeping properly hydrated, and maintaining the sodium-potassium balance.

Primary Objective 2: Maximize Muscular Definition and Tightness

Maximizing muscular definition and tightness is simply making sure every striation, every muscle, and the separation between the muscle groups is as visible and crisp as possible. Much of this is accomplished through minimizing extra cellular water retention by controlling four main factors: optimizing glycogen storage, minimizing glucose spill, avoiding dehydration, and maintaining the sodium-potassium balance.

Secondary Objective 1: Manage Vascularity

Vascularity is controlled by managing three factors: adequate hydration, proper sodium intake, and the regulation of substances in the bloodstream. Vascularity is not actively judged on a bodybuilding stage; it can enhance or detract from the look of a competitor depending on the division in which they are competing. The appearance of visible veins can enhance the look of a bodybuilder on stage, lending to a more extreme appearance. It is eye-catching and is usually a signal to the judges that a person is lean and full. However, for women in the bikini or figure divisions, vascularity can be a detriment. Bikini and figure do not call for an extreme look, so it is best to reduce vascularity for these divisions or at least not enhance it.

Secondary Objective 2: Create Consistency for Predictable Outcomes

You create consistency by eliminating unnecessary variables. Some of the best ways to do this are by avoiding gastrointestinal (GI) tract issues and food allergies through eating only familiar foods and avoiding inaccurate measurements by not changing food sources too much.

The results of a peak week should be predictable. You should not have to cross your fingers and hope that it works. A proper peak week should be measurable, predictable, and repeatable. Create as much consistency as possible to reduce unnecessary risks and make the process more repeatable for future shows.

GI tract irritation and slight food allergies can come from eating unfamiliar foods. Often, people believe that magic foods make for the best peak week, while others tend to view their food choices as having no bearing at all on the outcome. The truth is that while food choices are not magic, they do indeed matter. If you have not eaten brown rice during the entire prep, it is not wise to add it in three days out from the show.

Another reason to stay with the same foods during every day of peak week is that food labels can be incredibly inaccurate. The U.S. Food and Drug Administration allows a 20 percent margin of error on food labels. This means that it is possible to eat a brand of cereal with a labeled caloric value 20 percent below the actual value. If you were to switch brands during peak week, the new brand label might list the caloric value 20 percent above the actual value. In this instance, you would be consuming 40 percent more calories even though the labels are the same. While this is an unlikely and extreme instance, this type of inconsistency can add up. Changing food during peak week is usually an unnecessary risk. After the show, you will be free to eat many foods that you have been wanting to try.

PEAK WEEK OBJECTIVE NONSTARTERS

These three objectives may seem simple enough, but as we will soon establish, many factors must be managed to achieve one's best look. The following are what we refer to as **peak week objective nonstarters**—objectives that set you up for failure before you even start.

Getting Leaner

Peak week is *not* for getting leaner. You should have lost all the body fat you need to lose going into peak week. If you have to choose between trying to peak properly or trying to get leaner, you will be better off just continuing to diet and get leaner. Better yet, pick a different show and give yourself more time.

Dropping Water

Peak week is *not* for dropping water. We will cover this in depth, but dropping water or dehydrating is not a goal.

Thinning the Skin

Thinning the skin is an absurd idea that needs to be abandoned. There is no way to effectively thin the skin. Going into peak week with the idea that skin thickness is an issue will lead to failure. If you think your skin is too thick, we are certain that you just have more fat to lose.

CARBOHYDRATES

We covered our prerequisites, brushed up on common terminology, and established clear objectives for peak week. Now we will get down to the nitty-gritty of peak week and begin learning about the many working parts of peak week. There is no better place to start than carbohydrates.

Carbohydrates, water, and sodium are the primary variables in an interconnected system of moving parts that we refer to as the **peaking network**. There are other parts to the peaking network, but carbohydrates, water, and sodium are the glue that hold everything together.

When talking about carbohydrates, we could go down a nearly endless rabbit hole discussing the various types, digestion, and metabolism of carbohydrates. However, this information is not always necessary to know to peak properly. Therefore, when it comes to carbohydrates, we cover the basics and the relevant details specifically related to peaking.

Types

Carbohydrate, or **carbs** for short, is a macronutrient found in various foods. Carbs are also referred to as **saccharides**, which can be divided into four groups: **monosaccharides**, **disaccharides**, **oligosaccharides**, and **polysaccharides**. Monosaccharides and disaccharides are smaller and have lower molecular weight and are commonly referred to as **sugar**. Monosaccharides are comprised of one sugar molecule (hence the prefix, **mono**) and disaccharides have two monosaccharides (hence the prefix, **di**). Common monosaccharides are glucose, fructose, ribose, and galactose. Common disaccharides include sucrose, which is table sugar, and lactose, which is the sugar found in milk.

Oligosaccharides and polysaccharides are **complex carbohydrates** because they are made of up more sugar molecules. Oligosaccharides typically have 3 to 7 monosaccharides, and polysaccharides contain more than 10.

Digestion

Carb digestion begins with our saliva. The enzyme **salivary amylase** kicks off the process. As we chew, this enzyme breaks the bonds between the sugar units of the various sugars and starches. This breaks down some carbs into smaller chains of glucose. Roughly only 5 percent of carbohydrates are broken down in the mouth. This is probably a good thing. If every carbohydrate we ate was fully broken down into glucose in our mouths, our teeth would probably rot out. The demand for dentists would be incredible, and you would probably be practicing dentistry rather than trying to be a bodybuilder! After the minimal digestion taking place in the mouth, the carbohydrates go to the stomach. In the stomach, no chemical digestion takes place, but there is some mechanical digestion from stomach contractions.

The carbohydrates then pass into the small intestine, where pancreatic amylase starts to break down the **dextrins** (polysaccharides) into sequentially smaller carbohydrate chains. While this is taking place, various enzymes also released by the intestinal cells break down the specific types of carbohydrates into singular sugar molecules. After carbohydrates are fully broken down into their most basic units, they can then be transported into the intestinal cells.

Transportation, Absorption, and Storage

Once carbohydrates reach the intestines, the monosaccharide units of glucose, fructose, and galactose are transported through the small intestine wall to the **portal vein** (the blood vessel that carries blood to the liver from the GI tract and spleen). The speed at which carbohydrates are absorbed can differ depending on whether proteins or fats were consumed as well. Fats and proteins slow the rate of absorption. Also, there are differences in the transportation paths of glucose, fructose, and galactose and where they end up. However, it is important to know that glucose is taken through the bloodstream to peripheral (noncentral) tissues. Excess glucose is stored as glycogen in the liver and muscle tissue.

So you may be asking, "Why do I need to know all this?" That is a valid question. Knowing the basics of carbohydrate types, digestion, transportation, absorption (also called **assimilation**), and storage is never a bad thing for a bodybuilder. However, the main takeaway of this is that digestion, transportation, and absorption take time. Competitors often try to carb up minutes before heading out to the stage. There is no time for all this digestion and assimilation. An effective carb-up needs to take place in the days before the show, not the minutes and hours before the show.

Role of Glycogen

In peaking discussions, you will frequently hear **glycogen** mentioned because it can greatly impact physique appearance. Glycogen is a polysaccharide that serves as the primary source of stored carbohydrates in the body. It is mostly stored in the muscle and liver cells. There are also small amounts of glycogen stored in the kidneys and the brain. For our purposes, though, we will primarily focus on the glycogen stored in the muscle tissue and liver.

Glycogen can provide an advantage to a bodybuilder by increasing muscle size and volume. A muscle packed full of glycogen will physically increase in size. Obviously, a bigger muscle is something that all bodybuilders want, so bodybuilders should try to completely fill their bodies' glycogen storage spaces without exceeding storage capacity. Eating more carbohydrates than the body can store in muscle tissue and the liver will result in spilling or spillover. When this happens, the additional glucose floats around outside the muscle cells, blurring muscle definition. Obviously, this is not a good thing. When carbing up, it is usually best to be slightly less filled rather than pushing things too hard and spilling. A slightly flat look will appear much more crisp and complete versus a slightly spilled one that looks puffy and blurry.

One final factor when considering glycogen is the supercompensation effect. Glycogen supercompensation is something that runners and other athletes have been taking advantage of for quite some time (4), and bodybuilders are no different. Always remember that the body strives for homeostasis, which is the tendency toward a stable equilibrium. This means that when you push your body in one direction, it typically corrects the imbalance as quickly as possible. It is like a pendulum; when you swing it one way, it swings back the other direction. Bodybuilders can use this advantage when carbing up. When the body is depleted of glycogen for roughly three to five days, glycogen storage capacity increases by about 10 to 20 percent. This means you can store more glycogen and be a bit fuller by depleting first (5). This is indeed a viable option for competing bodybuilders, but as we will see in the Peak Week Strategies section, this is not always the best option.

We will get deeper into peaking and carb-up strategies later in this chapter, but one thing to note (based on the authors' experience) is that the way carbs are loaded seems to make a difference in the look achieved. When carbohydrate levels are actively rising, the look tends to be fuller and more extreme. For example, say we have two competitors carbed up to 90 percent of full capacity. Now assume that the first competitor reached this point by coming up from 80 percent of his capacity while the second competitor reached this point by coming from 100 percent. In our experience, the competitor whose carbohydrates have been actively rising will have a bit fuller and tighter look. We cannot claim to know the mechanism behind this, but this is something we have witnessed through years of experience. It could be due to a miniature version of supercompensation effect in that intracellular fluids tend to be retained more effectively when coming from a more depleted state, but that is merely speculation.

Finally, while the amount of carbohydrate we consume influences glycogen levels, we see that water and sodium also play a role in this process. We cannot have proper storage of glycogen without the other factors in the peaking network.

WATER

Cutting water before a bodybuilding competition is practically a time-honored tradition. Walk into a bodybuilding show with a bottle of water and see all the stares you get. The other competitors will treat you as if you have already given up. Bodybuilders across the world still dehydrate, but is this practice effective?

What is causing this epidemic of aquaphobia in the bodybuilding community? The idea behind all this fear is that water under the skin blurs muscular definition; therefore, if you dehydrate yourself, there will be no water under the skin to blur definition. This seems like a nice, simple explanation, but the physiology is not quite so simple, and numerous problems stem from dehydrating to achieve a perfectly peaked physique.

Stored Glycogen to Water Ratio

In the carbohydrates section, we explained the importance of water for achieving maximum muscle fullness. Water stored with muscle glycogen provides fullness to our muscles. The ratio of glycogen to water is about one gram of glycogen for every 2.7 grams of water (2). However, it is possible to be even higher than that because some research shows it could be as high as a 1:3 or 1:4 ratio (3). That is just how important water is and how much it is responsible for filling the muscle.

Intracellular and Extracellular Fluid

Even though many people understand that the water stored with glycogen is responsible for muscle fullness, they believe they can trick the system and keep the water in the muscle while dehydrating the water not stored in the muscle. These people fail to understand that water balance within the human body is tightly regulated. The human body is roughly 60 percent water. Of this water, about 65 percent is **intracellular fluid** (ICF) located in compartments inside the body's cells, including muscle cells (figure 10.1). The other 35 percent is **extracellular fluid** (ECF) and is found outside the cells. Many people worry that this 35 percent of bodily fluid causes smoothness on stage. However, not all ECF is contained in spaces that would cause blurring of muscular definition. If we look at a rough breakdown of ECF, we see that 80 percent is called **interstitial fluid** and is found in the space between cells (called the **interstitial space**), while the other 20 percent is found elsewhere, such as blood plasma.

There are many misconceptions about how water is compartmentalized within the body. Advertising for commercial diuretics and persistent myths have given bodybuilders the impression that a layer of water underneath the skin hides striated muscle. However, if this was how water was stored underneath the skin, then we would see a lot of bodybuilders backstage simply poking themselves with a pin and draining the water out. Clearly this is not the case because there is not a layer of water underneath the skin.

While you do not need to know what it looks like under the skin to peak properly, peaking is not as simple as dropping water as many would have you believe. The human body is complex, and trying to selectively alter one area of it without altering other areas is impossible. Selective dehydration is not possible.

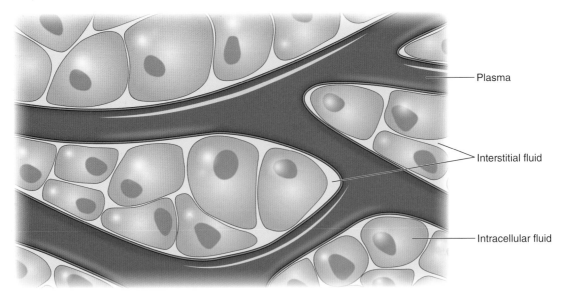

Figure 10.1   A closer look at interstitial fluid and intracellular fluid.

Interstitial Fluid

When it comes to extracellular fluid, the main area of concern for bodybuilders should be **interstitial fluid**. This is the fluid found in the interstitial space that can cause the blurring of muscular definition. It also contains various salts, hormones, and other **solutes** such as glucose, sodium, and potassium. What can you do to reduce the amount of interstitial fluid you hold? You cannot! Remember, the body tightly controls water compartments. However, there is no need to worry. The water balance of your body naturally works in your favor. Most fluid in your body is held in the intracellular compartments, which is where you want it because it provides fullness to your muscles. Plasma fluid is another area to hold water because it means more blood flow and a better pump.

You may be asking how people spill over if interstitial fluid is nothing to worry about. That is a good question. In this situation, water is not the problem; typically excess glucose (carbohydrates) is the problem. As we covered in the Carbohydrates section, your goal should be to fill the muscle with as much carbohydrate as possible. When you fill the muscle with glycogen, water follows. However, once the muscle tissue has reached maximum capacity, the glucose has nowhere else to go. In this case, the excess glucose will spill over and tend to float around in the interstitial fluid. When this happens, water follows the glucose in the interstitial space, and the amount of fluid in this space increases. Always remember that water follows solutes. Wherever there is glucose, sodium, or potassium, water will follow. So, we need to be sure that solutes are placed where we want them and in the amounts we want. If we do this, water can be kept high throughout peak week and will be stored where it should. Any excess water is simply expelled from the body through urination. This means that spilling and holding water—as most people think of it—is not caused by water intake but most commonly by too many carbohydrates.

An analogy can paint a clearer picture of why spilling over is the result of too many carbs rather than water. Pretend that your body is like a bathtub with the drain opened. When the faucet is turned on, water pours into the tub, but it drains out just as quickly. Now throw sponges (which represents glucose) into the tub. The water begins to stick (soak in) to the sponges in the tub but, as before, any excess water drains out. If we continue to throw more sponges into the tub with the faucet still on, more water will fill the sponges in the tub. However, if we throw so many sponges into the tub that they overfill the tub with the faucet still on, the water will start to spill over the top and end up all over the floor. In this scenario, the water being on was not the problem. The problem was that we tried to use more sponges than the tub could hold. Had we not breached the top of the tub with the sponges, the water would have never spilled over.

Spilling over occurs when we try to eat more carbohydrates than our bodies can store as glycogen. Once glycogen stores are filled, the excess carbs will spill out, and water will follow. Our goal should be to fill glycogen completely without exceeding our capacity. This will maximize ICF and minimize ECF.

With this knowledge, we must be like Goldilocks in our approach to carbing up. A carb-up that is too small will have you saying, "This carb-up left me too flat!" A carb-up that is too aggressive will leave you saying, "This carb-up left me spilled and blurry!" However, if you hit the right amount, you will be left saying, "This carb-up was juussst right."

As for water, we find that most people do well during peak week with a steady intake of 1 to 2.5 gallons (3.8-9.5 liters) per day, every day up until show day.

FAQ: Would you ever recommend that a competitor cut water during peak week?

In about 99 percent of cases, we do not recommend competitors cut water. The only case in which we might recommend that someone moderately cut water is if she is a bikini competitor who is too lean and too muscular for the bikini division. In this case, the goal of cutting water would be to make her look less lean and muscular in order to better fit the criteria of the bikini division. Everyone else should leave it in.

SODIUM-POTASSIUM BALANCE

While carbs and water are the main players in a proper peak week, sodium and potassium can be the icing on the cake. These are often misunderstood and underestimated factors in the peaking process. Some people massively adjust (often incorrectly) these variables while others say that you should not touch them. Which is correct? The truth is that you can enhance your look by manipulating sodium and potassium but doing so only slightly is often the best approach.

The fear of sodium before a show comes with the idea that sodium makes you hold water. This is true. As we covered in the last section, water follows solutes. Sodium makes you hold additional water, carbohydrates make you hold water, and potassium makes you hold water. However, the question should not be, "Am I holding water?" It should be, "Am I holding water in the right places?" Holding a higher than normal amount of water is a good thing if we are holding that water in compartments that will enhance the look we want.

For decades, bodybuilders have been cutting sodium before shows and loading up on potassium. While everyone seems to do it differently, usually people completely cut all additional sodium about three days out from the show and then begin either taking potassium supplements or carb loading by eating potatoes, which contain plenty of potassium. The myth of cutting sodium and increasing potassium most likely arose because sodium is found in large concentrations in the interstitial fluid, and potassium is found in large concentrations in the ICF (table 10.1). When hearing this, people say, "Aha! I knew I could reduce interstitial water! I will just cut sodium and load potassium, and all water will follow potassium into the cell because there will be no sodium to draw water to the interstitial space."

While this does appear to make sense, once again, it does not work that way in real life. The first thing we need to know about sodium and potassium is that they work together to control water balance in and out of the cells by the sodium-potassium (NA-K) pump. The problem is that the pump requires *both* sodium and potassium to operate correctly (figure 10.2).

The NA-K pump works by transporting two potassium ions *into* the cell while transporting three sodium ions *out* of the cell. Potassium cannot make it into the cell to provide more fullness

Table 10.1   Average Sodium and Potassium Concentrations

SOLUTE	SODIUM CONCENTRATION (MMOL/L)	POTASSIUM CONCENTRATION (MMOL/L)
Interstitial fluid	145	4.1
Intracellular fluid	12	150

Data from Lote (1).

without sodium. If you cut sodium, then the NA-K pump will stop working, and potassium will begin to pile up outside the cells and draw water to it. Once again, this leads to spilling.

Besides being an integral part of the proper functioning of the NA-K pump, sodium is also a contributor to facilitating glucose transport into the cell. As you can see in figure 10.2, sodium cycles into the cell with glucose and then cycles out of the cell as potassium makes its way in. This process continues over and over. If sodium were eliminated from this process, glucose would not make it into the cells efficiently and neither would potassium. When this happens, both potassium and glucose will begin to build up *outside* the cells. As they continue to float around outside the cells, water will follow. When water starts to accumulate outside the cells at abnormal levels, spilling happens yet again. Therefore, eliminating sodium is yet another way you can cause spill and a smoothing appearance to your physique. You must leave sodium in your diet to look your best!

In addition to proper intracellular and extracellular water balance, sodium also controls blood volume. Higher sodium intakes lead to greater blood volume, which leads to a greater pump, which leads to a bigger, fuller look. All great things!

With this knowledge, it should be clear that you should never cut sodium or load potassium in excessive amounts. We have found that a ratio of 3:1 to 5:1 of sodium to potassium work well for most people.

Unfortunately, we cannot tell you exactly how much carbs, water, sodium, and potassium you require during peak week. Each person has different requirements, but once you understand how the variables all interact with each other, you can try new and subtle combinations while avoiding disaster situations. If you are already looking great going into peak week (which you should be), then a conservative approach is always best when you are not sure what to do.

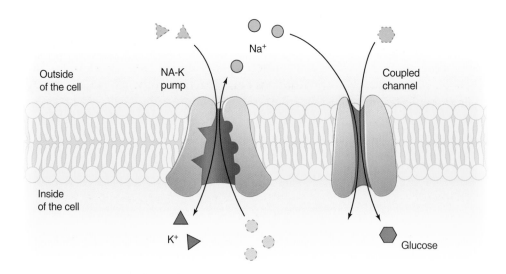

Figure 10.2   The sodium-potassium pump.

PEAKING NETWORK

If you ever wondered why so many bodybuilders seem to mess up the peak, all you need to do is look at figure 10.3. This chart clearly displays the needed components and their relationships for an effective peak. Most bodybuilders try to eliminate water and sodium, and they are effectively destroying any chance of ever coming in at their best.

The answer to effectively peaking lies largely within these components. Many people ask what to do about proteins and fats during peak week. This can change quite a bit based on what type of peak week strategy you employ. The strategy largely depends on your situation, body type, and division. Let us explore some of the best options.

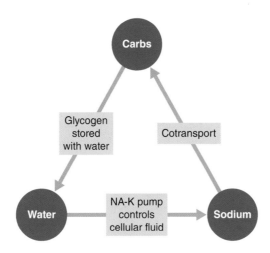

Figure 10.3   The peaking network: The relationship between carbs, water, and sodium.

PEAK WEEK STRATEGIES

Peak week strategies can be extremely confusing to those new to competition. While we covered a lot of information in the last section regarding carbs, water, and sodium, we did not cover how to structure these variables. This is where peak week strategies come into play. When it comes to peak week strategy and the information in this section, there are a few factors to consider.

► There is no right or wrong way to structure a peak week. Some peak week strategies are more appropriate for certain situations or certain people, but these are usually nuanced differences in results.

► The approaches are merely a guide, not a hard rule. While we list some of the most common structured setups, the combinations are practically endless. We are merely using our experience to provide a proper outline.

► Subtle changes to the variables are always more appropriate when you are less familiar with the process. If you have never tried a peaking strategy before, then be conservative with your changes, and, even better, practice it before show day.

► No peaking strategy should be rigid. When we work with our clients, we are constantly changing, adjusting, and adapting the plan during peak week. Do not be afraid to adjust variables on a day-to-day basis if you need to. Never be a slave to the plan.

Physique Management Peaking Strategies

If you are a novice or newer to peaking, we recommend using one of the **physique management peaking** strategies because they allow for the greatest day-to-day assessment and adjustments. With these peaking protocols, you can judge your physique each day and make judgment calls for the day based on how you look. Although you will have a general layout for how your week should progress, they are easily adjustable and safely executed because the changes are subtle.

It is important to note that all peak week structures are named after the stage of the week in which the carbohydrates are loaded.

Front-Load Peaking Protocol

As the name implies, the front-load peaking protocol has carbs loaded at the front of the week (figure 10.4). Typically, carbohydrates should be loaded on the Saturday and Sunday (possibly Monday as well, if needed) before a show. Carbs should be loaded over these two or three days to the point where a bit of spilling occurs. This ensures complete filling of available glycogen storage space. As the week progresses, taper carbs down to clean up the spillover. As the spill is cleaned up, definition and crispness improves. Typically, carbs should then be increased Friday before the show or on the morning of the show.

Protein and fat should be slightly lower on days when carbs are highest, but for the most part, they should stay rather steady with where intake was at during the entire contest prep. Keep water intake high and consistent throughout the week. Sodium should follow closely along the path of carbohydrates, with a bit more of an increase on Friday and again on show day.

The front-load peaking protocol is best for bikini and figure divisions. It is also great for beginner bodybuilders, or those less familiar with the peaking process or those who want a conservative and easy-to-execute peak week. This is the most conservative of all the peaking strategies and the option that has the least chance of something going wrong.

The primary advantage of this peaking strategy is safety, but it also creates a tight yet less extreme look perfect for bikini and figure. It can also create a good look for bodybuilders; however, it is just a slightly less full look when compared to some other peaking methods. This method is also useful for bodybuilders who show signs of insulin resistance because they blur when they carb up. It allows someone to carb up yet lets any blurring dissipate over the course of the week. In this instance, you may not want to bring carbohydrates up on Friday before the show. Instead, you would just continue to taper down.

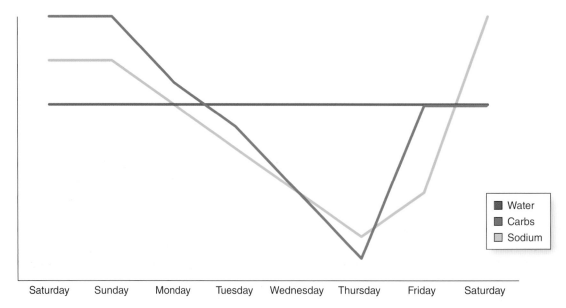

Figure 10.4 Front-load peaking protocol.

Mid-Load Peaking Protocol

The mid-load peaking protocol typically begins with carbs lower at the beginning of the week (figure 10.5). Slowly build carbs as the week progresses, with carbohydrates hitting a high point on either Wednesday or Thursday. With this strategy, you may want to see only slight spilling when you load up; then you can use Friday, or Thursday and Friday, to then taper carbohydrates, clean up the spill, and sharpen up.

Protein and fat should be slightly lower on days when carbs are highest, but for the most part, they should stay steady with where intake was at during the entire contest prep. Keep water intake high and consistent throughout the week. Sodium should track closely with carbohydrate intake, with a possible increase on Friday as well as on show day.

The mid-load peaking protocol is best for bikini, figure, and men's physique divisions. It is also great for beginner bodybuilders, bodybuilders who are less familiar with the peaking process, or those who want a conservative and easy-to-execute peak week. While this is not as conservative as the front-load protocol, it is still conservative and easy to execute.

The primary advantage of this peaking strategy is safety, and it tends to create a bit more fullness than a front-load peak. Mid-load peaking works well for bikini and figure competitors who need additional fullness come show day. This peaking method is also useful for bodybuilders who show signs of insulin resistance because they blur when carbing up. It allows someone to carb up and lets any blurring dissipate over the day or two before the show, when carbs are tapered.

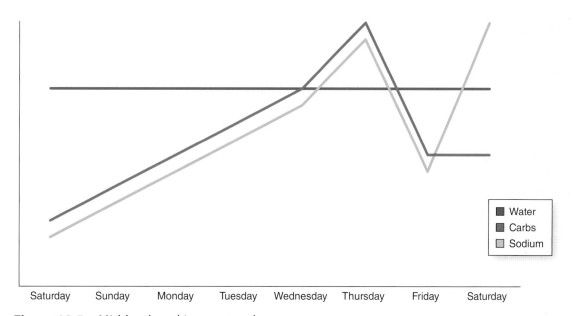

Figure 10.5 Mid-load peaking protocol.

Slow Back-Load Peaking Protocol

Slow back-load peaking begins with carbs low at the beginning of the week (figure 10.6). As you slowly increase carbs as the week progresses, you will notice your physique getting tighter and filling out a bit more each day. With this peaking strategy, you should never aim to spill at any point during the week. Your goal is to hit your highest carbohydrate intake on Friday. If at any point during the week you notice that you are starting to spill over, taper carbs downward for the remaining days, and in effect you will turn it into a mid-load peak.

Protein and fat should be slightly lower on days when carbs are highest, but for the most part, they should stay rather steady with the same intake as the rest of contest prep. Keep water intake high and consistent throughout the week. Sodium should track rather closely with carbohydrate intake, with a possible increase on Friday as well as show day.

The slow back-load peaking protocol is a versatile peaking strategy for all divisions. In divisions where a subtler look is required (bikini and figure), carbohydrates should be increased more subtly, and in divisions where a more extreme look is required (bodybuilding and physique), a more drastic carbohydrate increase looks best.

This peaking strategy is a bit harder to execute than a front- or mid-load as you aim to perfectly predict your highest carb intake on the day before the show. If you guess wrong, it could leave you too flat on show day or spilled if you are too aggressive. However, if done correctly, this is an excellent peaking strategy that can offer a variety of looks depending on how drastically carbohydrates are increased. Since this peaking strategy is a bit more risky than a front-load or mid-load, it may not be a bad idea to run through a mock peak week with it if you are early to ensure that you know what to expect during peak week.

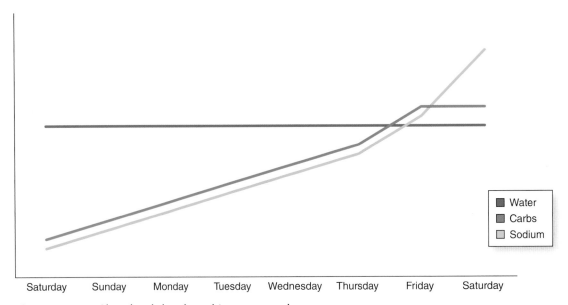

Figure 10.6 Slow back-load peaking protocol.

Glycogen Supercompensation Peaking Strategies

As the name implies, **glycogen supercompensation peaking** involves trying to take advantage of the supercompensation effect seen when carbohydrates are depleted. Initially, many bodybuilders are drawn to these forms of peaking. However, any peaking strategy that employs more drastic changes and measures also has a greater chance of going wrong. With physique management peaking strategies, you can use subtle changes and day-to-day analysis to ease into the look that you want. With glycogen supercompensation peaking, you typically get one chance to get it right, and if you are wrong, then things will not look good on show day. While these peaking methods are effective, you absolutely must know what you are doing and have practiced them.

Back-Load Peaking Protocol

Back-load peaking typically begins with a carbohydrate deplete phase (figure 10.7). Remember that glycogen depleting is the most effective when it is set up as a carbohydrate deplete, not a calorie deplete. To set up a proper deplete, calories should be within 200 calories of where your dieting intake was. For example, if you had finished your contest prep on 2,000 calories per day, then your deplete should likely be 1,800 to 2,200 calories per day. If you feel you could be a little leaner, you should set your caloric intake 200 calories below your normal dieting amount. If you feel that you are lean enough, then you can set your caloric intake exactly where you have been dieting or even slightly above. The amount of carbohydrates eaten during a deplete phase depends largely on the individual. However, we have noticed that most people need to deplete

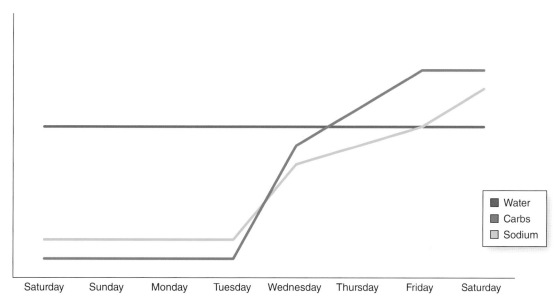

Figure 10.7   Back-load peaking protocol.

with carbohydrates in the range of 50 to 100 grams per day. Once carbohydrate intake has been set, protein and fat intakes should be increased to reach calorie goals for the day.

A deplete phase should not run too long or you risk muscle loss, flattening out so much that you cannot fully refill glycogen levels by show day, or both. However, the deplete phase needs to be long enough to fully deplete glycogen stores. Ideally, you want the phase to be about three or four days long.

Once you have fully depleted, the carb-up should begin either Wednesday or Thursday before the show and extend through Friday. While some people have two or three days of the same carbohydrate intake, we have found that building carbs each day works well as long as the carb increase is aggressive. The amount of carbohydrates you can handle during these carbohydrate-loading days varies drastically from person to person. For this reason, we recommend practicing this peaking style before using it for an actual contest. When executed properly, however, back-load peaking can be effective.

As mentioned, during the deplete phase, protein and fat intakes should be higher to bring calorie levels where needed. However, during the loading days, protein and fat intakes should be dropped to a slightly lower intake than what was normal during the entirety of contest prep. Water intake should be kept high and consistent throughout the week. Sodium should track rather closely with carbohydrate intake.

The back-load peaking protocol is best for men's and women's bodybuilding, women's physique, and figure competitors who are undersized for their divisions. This strategy tends to produce more drastic looks suitable for divisions that require a more extreme look. Do not run this peaking strategy unless you are very lean. If you still have weight to lose, then you are better off going with one of the physique management peaking strategies.

This peaking strategy increases the size of muscles due to the supercompensation effect; however, the more extreme nature of the strategy means more risk. Generally, the more working parts of the peak week, and the greater the fluctuations in carbs and sodium, the more chances there will be for error. Practice this style of peaking before trying it for a real show.

Back-Load Peaking With Cleanup Day Protocol

Back-load peaking with a cleanup day works like a back-load peak, but it is a bit more forgiving (figure 10.8). This method will also begin with a carbohydrate deplete phase. As with the back-load peaking protocol, it is important to understand that glycogen depletion is more effective as a carbohydrate deplete and not a calorie deplete, and calories should be within 200 of contest prep calories. Those who need to be a little leaner can set calories 200 under their normal amounts, but if body fat is already acceptable, calories can be kept at the same level or even slightly above. The amount of carbohydrates eaten during a deplete phase depends largely on the individual, but most people need to deplete with about 50 to 100 grams of carbohydrates per day. Be sure to allow protein and fat intake to increase to reach the needed daily caloric intake.

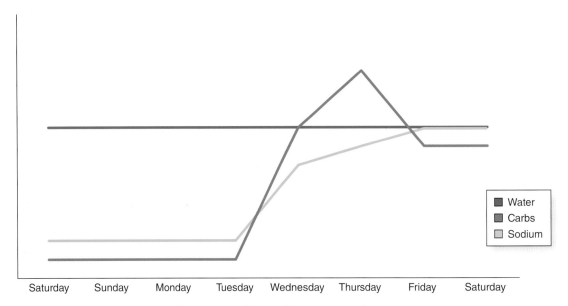

Figure 10.8   Back-load with cleanup day peaking protocol.

A deplete phase should not be too long or muscle may be lost, or you take the chance that you may flatten out so much that glycogen levels cannot be refilled by show day. Despite that risk, the deplete phase needs to be long enough (3-4 days) to fully deplete glycogen stores. After a full depletion, the carb-up should begin on Tuesday or Wednesday and extend through Thursday. Building carbs each day is an effective approach (if the increase is aggressive), although the amount of carbohydrates that a person can tolerate varies.

The primary difference between this peak week protocol and the back-load peaking protocol is that, rather than continuing to build carbohydrates into the show, on the day before the show, pull carbohydrate intake back a bit and clean up any spilling that may have occurred. This way, you can take full advantage of glycogen supercompensation while having a buffer day to fix any mistakes made by carbing up too aggressively. Note, though, that when carbohydrates are actively rising, your physique will look a bit fuller. You may see a bit more fullness with a back-load peaking protocol, but the difference will be small.

Protein and fat intakes should be higher during the deplete phase to bring the day's caloric intake up to where it needs to be, but during the loading days, protein and fat intake should be slightly lower than their levels during contest prep. Keep water intake high and consistent throughout the week, and changes in sodium intake should follow the changes in carbohydrate intake.

The back-load with cleanup day peaking protocol is best for men's and women's bodybuilding, women's physique, and figure competitors who are undersized for their divisions. This protocol produces a more extreme look for the divisions that require it. Beware, though; this protocol is not recommended for those who still need to lose body fat. Those competitors should follow one of the physique management peaking strategies.

Rapid Back-Load Peaking Protocol

The rapid back-load peaking strategy was developed in 2010 by the coauthor, Cliff Wilson. When Cliff noticed the phenomenon that competitors tended to look fuller and more extreme when carbohydrates were more drastically rising, it seemed only natural to see whether the entire carb-up could be executed in a single day to create the greatest possible fullness. Although this peaking strategy can produce extreme results, it is extremely difficult to execute unless you know exactly what you are doing.

The rapid back-load peaking protocol is best for men's and women's bodybuilding. This peaking strategy produces the most drastic look, so it is only recommended for a bodybuilder. It is not appropriate for any other division.

The protocol begins by slightly increasing carbohydrates over a one- or two-day period (figure 10.9). The purpose of this is to avoid going into the deplete phase too flat. You do not want to be fully carbed up to begin the deplete, but you also do not want to be flat. A good guideline is having two days where carbs and calories are like what you would do on your typical refeed days during contest prep.

After the two days of increased carbs, you will enter a four- to five-day deplete phase. Four days of depleting is usually best, which would mean depleting Monday-Thursday if the show is on Saturday. Remember that glycogen depletion is the most effective when it is set up as a carbohydrate deplete, not a calorie deplete. To set up a proper deplete, calories should be within a 200-calorie range above or below what you were consuming while dieting. If you feel you could be a little leaner, then place your intake 200 calories below your normal dieting amount. If you feel that you are lean enough, then you can set them exactly where you have been dieting or even slightly above.

The amount of carbohydrates to eat during the depletion phase is specific to the person, but most people need to deplete with carbohydrates in the range of 40 to 80 grams per day for a rapid back-load peak. After carbohydrate intake has been set, protein and fat intakes should be increased to reach calorie goals for the day.

After the carbohydrate deplete phase, the carbohydrate-loading phase should begin on the day before the show. The amount of carbohydrates that someone should consume varies based on many factors. However, we have found that most female competitors will do well consuming 4.8 to 6.5 grams of carbohydrates per pound of body weight (10.56-14.3 g of carbohydrates per kg). Most male competitors will do well consuming between 5.5 and 7.4 grams of carbohydrates per pound (12.1-16.28 g per kg) of body weight. Some people could fall outside of these ranges, but most people fall within them. When deciding your carb-up amount, always err on the side of caution by starting lower with your estimation.

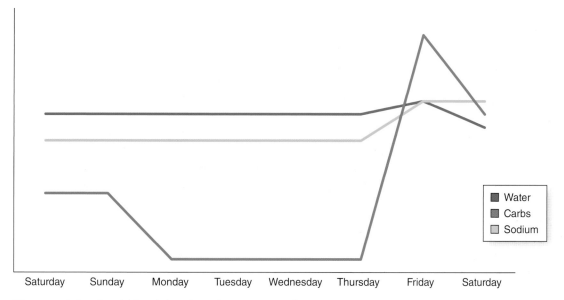

Figure 10.9 Rapid back-load peaking protocol.

We advise competitors to wake up early on carb-up day to begin eating. The carbohydrate-loading requirements mean that many people should consume between 700 to 1,300 grams of carbohydrates in a single day. Because the intake is so high, waking up early allows the carbs to be spread more evenly across the day without digestive distress. Consume faster-digesting carbohydrates earlier in the day, and as the loading day progresses, transition to slower-digesting carbohydrate sources.

Water intake over the week during a rapid back-load should be consistently high throughout the week, with only a slight increase on the carbohydrates loading day. Sodium should similarly be kept consistently high throughout the entire week. Most other peaking strategies do well to have sodium track upward or downward with carbohydrates, but this peaking style is best with consistent sodium levels with only a slight increase on the loading day.

As mentioned, during the deplete phase, protein and fat intakes should be higher to bring calorie levels where needed. During the load day, protein and fat intake should be minimal. Protein and fat intake should be reserved to whatever trace amounts are contained within the carbohydrate-loading foods you are consuming that day.

This peaking strategy is absolutely the most difficult one to execute. Because all carbohydrate loading is done in one day, there is little margin for error. By the time you can tell if you have carbed up properly, it is too late to change anything. Practice this form of peaking before trying it in an actual show day situation.

LEARNING YOUR LOAD LOOK AND CHOOSING A PEAKING STRATEGY

One final consideration when choosing a peak week strategy is something called your load look. Cliff coined this phrase some time ago to describe how someone looks while they are carb loaded and the day or so after they are carb loaded. Some people tend to have a tight load look. This means that while they are in the process of being carb loaded—and in the period after the load—they seem to look sharper, and the skin looks more tightly wrapped around the muscle. Even if they spill over slightly, the skin still may look tight. This is also usually accompanied by a lot of vascularity. On the other hand, some people have a soft load look. This means that when they are carb loading, they get blurry and soft or possibly even bloated around the midsection. People with a soft load look often find they stay blurry for a day or two and are sharpest about one to three days after carb load.

While we cannot claim to know with certainty the reason some people have different load looks, we speculate that it is due to varied levels of insulin sensitivity between individuals or that some people do not synthesize glycogen as quickly as others. For people with a soft load look, glucose may be floating around in the interstitial spaces for a while before being stored as muscle glycogen (thereby drawing water and causing blurring).

Regardless, learn your own individual load look before peak week. If you have a tight load look, it would be better to have carbs coming up more aggressively into show day. If you have a soft load look, it would be wise to choose a peaking strategy where your more aggressive loading is finished one to three days before the show. Knowing your load look helps you manage your physique on show day, as we will cover in the Managing Your Physique on Show Day section.

PEAK WEEK TRAINING

Competitors often incorrectly handle training during peak week. Typically, during the final week, motivation is at an all-time high. The excitement of the show usually results in energy and motivation levels that are higher than they have been in months. As a result, many competitors tend to train much harder during the final week. They lift heavier loads and perform a greater volume of work.

While this feels natural and good to lift more intensely when energy levels are high, it is the opposite of what you would want during peak week. By the time peak week has arrived, most of your hard work is over. At this stage, no new muscle is built. While the primary goal with your training during contest prep is to build and maintain muscle tissue, the goal during peak week shifts to facilitating proper glycogen storage, allowing for better recovery, and ensuring you are not sore on show day. Reducing the intensity and volume of training during peak week can reduce inflammation and create a slightly sharper look.

It may not feel particularly glamorous or exciting, but training during peak week needs to be rather boring and uneventful. There are a variety of ways to plan your training during peak week. Examples to follow for physique management peaking protocols and glycogen supercompensation peaking protocols are found in tables 10.2 and 10.3, respectively.

Table 10.2   Peak Week Training Plan for Physique Management Peaking Strategies

SATURDAY	SUNDAY	MONDAY	TUESDAY	WEDNESDAY	THURSDAY	FRIDAY	SHOW DAY
Off	Off	Legs	Back and biceps	Chest and triceps	Delts, traps, and abs	Whole-body circuit	—
—	—	75%-80% of normal volume and intensity	75%-80% of normal volume and intensity	75%-80% of normal volume and intensity	75%-80% of normal volume and intensity	50%-60% of normal volume and intensity	—
—	—	8-12 rep range	8-12 rep range	8-12 rep range	8-12 rep range	8-15 rep range	—

Table 10.3   Peak Week Training Plan for Glycogen Supercompensation Peaking Strategies

SATURDAY	SUNDAY	MONDAY	TUESDAY	WEDNESDAY	THURSDAY	FRIDAY	SHOW DAY
Off	Off	Legs	Back and biceps	Chest and triceps	Delts, traps, and abs	Whole-body circuit	—
—	—	75%-85% of normal volume and intensity	75%-85% of normal volume and intensity	75%-85% of normal volume and intensity	75%-85% of normal volume and intensity	50%-60% of normal volume and intensity	—
—	—	10-20 rep range	10-20 rep range	10-20 rep range	10-20 rep range	10-20 rep range	—

PEAK WEEK CARDIO

The cardio needed during peak week varies depending on the person. However, much like peak week training, the goal should be to try and reduce the intensity and duration of what you have been performing to allow for greater recovery. A few guidelines include the following:

- ► Avoid high-intensity interval training (HIIT) cardio during the final week. This is too intense and can impede recovery.
- ► Aim to reduce current cardio levels and taper as the week progresses. If possible, try to minimize cardio in the final one or two days before the show.
- ► Do not do new types of cardio during peak week. Stick with familiar modes of cardio so that soreness is not an issue.
- ► Cardio may need to be higher on deplete days, but aim to not have it any higher than what was common during prep.

MANAGING YOUR PHYSIQUE ON SHOW DAY

The big day is finally here! Maybe you nailed your peak week, maybe you did not, or maybe you are close but could be better. Are there things you can do in the final hours to make yourself better? Yes! Show-day nutrition often leads to more questions than answers, however. Let us clarify what to do, starting with the morning of the show.

Choose Your Food

Before show day arrives, plan what foods you need to eat to meet your macronutrient requirements. We recommend avoiding high-residue foods—foods higher in fiber and harder to digest—on show day. For example, this means avoiding vegetables because they often do not digest very efficiently and are more likely to cause bloating. Instead, eat light, easily digested foods that are low in fiber.

We also recommend keeping protein intake to just a few bites of chicken or beef with each meal or a small protein shake with a meal or two. This is also to avoid bloating on show day because protein is harder to digest. You do not need protein on show day; it does not serve any purpose, so there is no sense in forcing yourself to eat a lot of chicken, like you would on most other days.

Assess Your Physique

The first thing you need to do on show day is wake up early enough to assess your physique. Competitors often wake up only a few hours before the show. The big issue with this is that there is not enough time to create positive changes for your physique. If you are just a little bit off with your peak, you will want some time to correct the situation and get even better. The more certain you are that you nail your peak, the later you can wake up. We recommend waking up about six to six and a half hours before prejudging to assess your physique and begin adjustments. If you are certain you will nail your peak, you can wake up four to five hours before prejudging.

Get a Light Pump

After you have assessed your physique and determined if you are flat, spilled, or spot on, we recommend you get in a light pump session at home or in the hotel room. It does not need to be anything too involved; usually a light pump with some resistance bands, along with some push-ups, will be plenty. The purpose of this pump is twofold: it lets you see how you look with increased blood flow so you can further assess your status (sometimes it can be hard to tell right after you wake up), and it will facilitate improved glycogen storage of the carbohydrates you will eat in the morning. Remember, on show day, time is of the essence since carbs you eat do not convert to glycogen immediately. This pump should only be about 15 to 20 minutes long. What you do after the pump will depend largely on how you look.

If You Are Flat

If you woke up and are looking flat, it might be a good idea to start the day with some sort of liquid carb source such as Gatorade or a glucose drink. The carbs will get through your system and assimilate as quickly as possible. After that, you should try to eat every hour or hour and a half with quickly digested carb sources. You may also want to add a little sodium to help assimilate carbs. During this process, check your physique often. Once you see yourself starting to fill out, start slowing down your feeding. Carbs will not change your physique immediately. Give it a few hours to start taking effect, and do not carb up too aggressively. Remember that it is better to be a little flat rather than spilled.

It is also important to recall what your specific load look is. If you are a bit flat but have a soft load look, then you may be better off just leaving carbs moderate for show day, focusing on bringing fats up to preserve what you have and concentrating on staying tight rather than softening due to overzealous carbing up. If you have a tight load look, then you are likely be able to carb up more aggressively knowing that it only makes you tighter.

Water on show day is simple. You should aim to drink about 12 ounces (355 mL) of water with each meal. You can drink more if you are thirsty. You *need* water on show day to keep shuttling those carbs into your muscle tissue. You should not let yourself get thirsty. However, on show day, there is no reason to force water intake either.

If You Are Spilled

Hopefully you are not spilled on show day. We have said repeatedly that it is better to be flat than spilled. However, in real life, spilling happens. If you wake up and think you are a bit spilled, we recommend keeping food intake very low or possibly even having no food after your pump. If you are spilled over, it is because you have eaten too many carbohydrates the previous days. Therefore, you do not want to add more to your system. Instead, you want to use the glucose currently floating around in the subcutaneous areas.

We recommend eating only one or two very small meals before stage time and performing three or four small pump sessions in the hours before stage. These small pump sessions will continue to use some excess glucose and sharpen you up a bit before the stage. Typically, spilling over will take a day or two to correct; however, this is something you can do to help the situation.

Recommendations for water intake are the same as if you were flat; about 12 ounces (355 mL) with each meal (more if you are thirsty, but do not force it).

If You Are Spot On

If you wake up the morning of the show and look perfect, congrats! After your pump session, you should eat a small meal of moderate-high carbohydrates, low protein, and moderate fats. Do this every one and a half hours or so to maintain your physique. Stick with easily digested whole-food carb sources and about 12 ounces (355 mL) of water with each meal. You can drink more if you are thirsty, but there is no need to force water intake either.

The Final Minutes

In the final minutes before going on stage, there is still enough time to change your physique. Here are a few tactics that can help you make some last-minute improvements.

► *Sodium:* Sodium can enhance vascularity and a pump, which is a nice finishing touch to an already great-looking physique. About 45 to 60 minutes before stage time, a timely dose of 500 to 2000 milligrams (about 1/4-1 tsp of table salt) will work wonders for improving your pump and vascularity. Women, those in divisions requiring a less extreme look, and those with low sodium tolerance should stay on the lower end of that range.

► *Caffeine:* Caffeine will help with alertness on stage and ultimately just help you feel more energized, and it can also help you work up a bit of a sweat before the stage. People often tend to look a bit better after they have worked up a bit of a sweat.

► *Sugar:* Much like sodium, sugar enhances vascularity. Competitors once thought the key to vascularity was to drink red wine before the stage. However, there is nothing magical about red wine. The alcohol hitting the bloodstream caused veins to pop out. Any substance in the bloodstream causes increased vascularity. This means sodium, glucose, amino acids, alcohol, and so on will all cause your veins to protrude if they are flooding your bloodstream. We do not recommend using alcohol, but sodium and sugar are great choices. A quick dose of 20 to 50 grams of sugar about 20 to 30 minutes before stage can have a big effect.

FAQ: What if I mistime my sodium, sugar, and pump up backstage, and I am too early?

Judging the timing of when you are going on stage exactly can be difficult. It is usually better to do everything early rather than late. If you find that you pumped up too early, this is OK. All you must do is stop pumping for a few minutes, and then you can simply pump again. This will not cause you to flatten out, assuming you carbed up properly.

THE PERFECT PEAK?

We need to bring it all together with the knowledge that peaking is truly a combination of an art and science. Learning to peak properly is never as easy as putting together a formula that will work the same way every time. Peaking properly is not as simple as saying that a peak weak was a total success or a complete failure. Most often, you will always leave each peak week feeling you could have been fuller, tighter, bigger, and so on. Just remember that peaking is an ever-evolving process. You learn something new each time you do it. Experiment, practice, and always err on the side of conservatism come show day. If you do this, you will find yourself getting better and better while leaving others wondering what your secret is.

Take-Home Points

- ▶ To effectively peak, you *must* be lean!
- ▶ Carbohydrates, water, and sodium work together to create a full and tight look.
- ▶ Cutting out water while carbing up can cause blurring of definition and a softening of the physique.
- ▶ Removing sodium during peak week can cause spilling and a lack of pump.
- ▶ Many effective peaking strategies can be used to bring your best on show day.
- ▶ Peaking is a combination of an art and science and is perfected through a lot of trial and error.

Contest Weekend: Strategizing for Success

It does not matter what division you are competing in or the reasons you are competing. You have spent years training to build the necessary muscle to compete on a bodybuilding stage, and you have spent months dieting, training, and doing your cardio to get lean enough. You have endured hunger, fatigue, and deprivation to get to this day. You have made it further in this process than most people could ever imagine. The day is yours to enjoy. Hopefully, you have also had some extra carbohydrates during peak week to fill out a bit more in the days leading up to the show. Show day is the time to reveal the result of your hard work!

FOCUS ON WHAT YOU CAN CONTROL

For first-time competitors, show day can be an incredibly stressful experience filled with many unknowns. All competitors worry they may not place high. However, contest placing is based on three factors: how you look, who else shows up, and what the judges are looking for that day.

You have no control over who else is competing that day. A person with a high-level physique may win overall in one show and barely make top five in the next show simply based on whom they are standing with onstage.

In addition, what the judges are looking for may differ from one show to the next or even between judges within the same show. A competitive class won by a one-point decision may go the other way with a different judging panel.

Rather than stressing about factors you cannot control, focus on the one thing you have complete control over: how you look onstage. If you have applied the advice provided in this book, you should be able to step onstage looking your best.

Show day can feel overwhelming, even for seasoned competitors who are in their best shape ever. It can seem like there are so many details to keep straight. To complicate things further, the details may differ from show to show. This chapter will provide guidelines for show day so that you are prepared and can approach the day relaxed.

THE DAY BEFORE THE SHOW

The to-do list of a competition typically begins on the day before the show. Although each show schedule may differ, several appointments and meetings are usually held the day before the show. Competitors who are traveling to a show need to plan to arrive the day prior in most circumstances.

Check-In

To keep things running efficiently on show day, it is common to have a competitor check-in the day prior. This is when a competitor picks up his or her competitor number, drops off posing music, picks up a goodie bag (if provided by the contest sponsors), and has a chance to ask the promoter any last-minute questions.

If information about class order or class size is not provided, we recommend asking the promoter. Knowing the order of classes for show day can help you to properly time your peak so you look your best when it is time to step onstage with your class. It can also give you an idea of how much time you will have on show day.

Tanning

There are many different tanning options for competitors. Those who choose to be sprayed by a tanning service associated with the show will likely have an appointment the day before the show to apply the first coat of tan. An additional coat (or coats) will also be added on show day.

Competitors who have fair skin and are doing their own tans should do a base coat the day before the competition. In this situation, tan everything except your hands, feet, and face. Once the tan has dried, sleep in an old pair of sweatpants and a long-sleeved shirt to prevent smearing.

If you stay in a hotel, be sure to bring your own sheets and towels. Most tanning products rub off on the white sheets and towels provided by hotels. If this occurs, they will charge you for the damage.

Grooming

The day before a competition is a good time to take care of any last-minute grooming to save time on show day. This includes things like getting a haircut or doing a final removal of body hair. Females competing in bikini or figure need well-manicured nails.

Drug Testing

Drug-testing policies and procedures differ from show to show. However, most drug-tested competitions perform at least a portion of the drug test the day before competition. This may be a polygraph, urine test, or both. Urine samples may also be collected from competitors on show day. Consult the competitor information from your show for the drug-testing types and schedules at your competition.

Packing Your Bag for Show Day

On show day, you will be able to bring a bag with you backstage. This should include several items to help you to look your best onstage (see table 11.1). Preparing this bag early helps reduce your stress on show day.

Essential Items

The must-haves in your show-day bag include everything you will wear onstage: posing suit, shoes (for figure and bikini divisions), hair and makeup products, tan and oil products, and jewelry (for figure and bikini divisions). Have your food and water for the day to ensure that you stay on track with your peak plan. Make sure to bring towels to clean up any mess you make with your tan and oil. If your posing music was not collected at check-in, bring it with you on show day. Even if your posing music has been collected before show day, bring a backup copy.

Table 11.1   Show-Day Bag Items

ESSENTIAL ITEMS	OPTIONAL ITEMS
Posing suit	Resistance bands (to pump up)
Shoes (for figure and bikini divisions)	Mirror
Tanning and oil (or glaze) products	Extra posing suit
Hair and makeup products (if necessary)	Scissors, superglue, or double-stick tape
Jewelry (for figure and bikini divisions)	Bikini Bite
Food	Space heater and extension cord
Water	Cell phone charger
Towels	Blanket and pillow
Posing music (including a backup copy)	Plastic cup (women)

Optional Items

Several other items may not be essential for show day but may be helpful to have in your bag. Resistance bands to pump up are on the top of this list. Although most shows have weights backstage for you to pump up with before going out, equipment can be limited, and the pump-up area can be crowded. It is much easier to bring along some of your own resistance bands to use. Similarly, most shows have some mirrors backstage, but space in front of one can be crowded, so it be can helpful to bring your own mirror if you have one.

Plan for the worst when it comes to your suit. Things such as scissors, superglue, and double-stick tape can avert a suit crisis. If you have an extra suit, put it in your bag as a backup. Some competitors also find that the suit does not fit or stick where they would like. Bikini Bite is necessary to stick your suit to you to prevent any wardrobe malfunctions onstage.

The remaining optional items are needed because you will likely be sitting around and waiting a while on show day. Things such as a blanket and pillow to get comfortable, a small space heater to stay warm (often it is cold backstage!), and your cell phone charger may make the wait more pleasant. Finally, females may want to consider bringing a plastic cup with a hole in the bottom for the restroom so that you do not have to sit down and ruin your tan. It may be advisable to put toilet paper in the bowl before going to the bathroom to prevent water splatters that would ruin your tan.

SHOW DAY

The day has finally come! In this section we will cover a show day schedule that is somewhat typical. However, there can be variations in the show day schedule and timing, so be sure to consult your specific show information or ask the show promoter any questions that you have so that you know what to expect.

Competitors Meeting

Contest day typically begins with a competitors meeting. During this meeting, the show promoter will go over last-minute details, such as class order, number of competitors in each class, expectations for posing and sportsmanship, and any other last-minute information that competitors may need for the day.

If competitors in bikini, figure, and men's physique are not clear on the expectations for the T-walk, ask the show promoter at this meeting. Each show may do things a bit differently in the T-walk and individual presentation. Odds are, other competitors have the same questions.

Preparation for the Stage

After the competitors meeting, there is time before the prejudging to finish preparing for the stage. This is when you can finish your hair, makeup, and tan. Before stepping onstage, apply a glaze or oil, based on the tanning product you used.

Also, be sure to take time to relax and meet other competitors. Although competing can be stressful, and you will ultimately be compared against the others, everyone backstage is in the same position. Other competitors will help you out or answer your questions if you need something. Be sure to return the favor if needed. Most competitors backstage are supportive of each other and consequently have made several new friendships through competing.

Before stepping onstage, you will also want to briefly pump. This helps increase fluid in the muscle and results in looking larger and more vascular onstage. In general, it is best to pump the upper body with light weights or bands; for the lower body, stick to minimal pumping using just your body weight. Competitors in divisions that require more muscularity and vascularity need to pump more than those that do not. Additionally, competitors who are borderline too big or too vascular for their division may want to back off on pumping to not appear excessively muscular or vascular for the division.

FAQ: How ready should I be when I arrive at the venue on show day?

This is a hard question to answer because there is not a one-size-fits-all norm. It depends on how much time you have before your class, how much prep time you need, and your preferences. For example, a figure or bikini competitor who needs her hair, makeup, and tan done typically needs a good chunk of this completed before arriving at the venue, especially if her class is early in the show order. However, a men's bodybuilder competing in one of the last classes at a large show can typically arrive with only a base coat of tan and have plenty of time. It will be best to get an idea of how much time you have in advance and plan your show day schedule to give yourself plenty of time to get ready.

Prejudging

Prejudging is when most judging is completed. During prejudging, competitors come out onstage with the class. Competitors are positioned in a line and asked to complete the mandatory poses for their division (see chapter 8).

The judges often move competitors around the stage to make sure they can compare certain competitors next to each other and allow everyone to get a fair look. In general, being moved toward the middle of the stage is a good thing because it means they are against the top competitors in the class. Being moved *away* from the center is usually not a good thing, but this is not always the case because several sanctions have moved away from this style of judging. Instead, they move competitors around randomly onstage to allow each to get a fair look.

In large classes, judges may do callouts to compare smaller groups of competitors at a time. During callouts, the competitors being compared stand on the judging line while the other competitors not in the callout will be off to the back of the stage. If you are in the back of the stage, be sure to stay tight. Even if the judges are not directly comparing you, assume their eyes are on you. In general, the first callouts are the top competitors in the class; however, this is not always the case.

Some sanctions also have competitors perform T-walks during prejudging; however, this may differ between sanctions and even shows within the same sanction. Be sure to ask questions and be aware of what is required of your class during prejudging if it is not clear.

FAQ: Can I go out to eat after prejudging?

After prejudging, most shows are done judging you. However, if you feel you may win your class, then you should not go out to eat because you may need to compete in the overall competition and will be judged against the other class winners. It is better to stay on your plan.

We have seen situations where competitors were marked down due to looking significantly worse at night. When in doubt, stay consistent with your plan until after you come offstage at the night show.

Night Show

The night show is a much more relaxed atmosphere than prejudging. In general, all the judging is done (aside from overalls) at that point. However, if a competitor arrives at the night show looking significantly worse than at prejudging, he or she may be moved down a few places. Stick with your meal plan between shows, saving any treats until after the night show.

During the night show, competitors typically do their posing routines and receive their awards. In general, the crowd at the night show is larger. It is also when competitors' family and friends get to see them onstage since most noncompetitors may not get much out of prejudging.

Competitors who win divisions that have more than one class will also compete in the overall at the night show. For example, if there are three open bodybuilding classes, the winners of each of these classes will be compared, like prejudging. Ultimately, the winner will be awarded the overall champion. In larger pro qualifying competitions, the overall winner will also be awarded a pro card.

Live Judging

Many shows are beginning to move away from the traditional style of prejudging with a gap of downtime before the night show. Live-judged shows are becoming more common and are meant to be friendlier for competitors and their families and friends.

During a live-judged show, a competitor's class comes onstage for prejudging as usual. However, following the class comparisons, competitors will immediately perform their posing routines, during which time scores are tallied. Following the posing routines, awards are handed out. Many competitors and spectators who have experienced live-judged shows have positive things to say about their experience. As a result, this show format is increasing in popularity and the prevalence likely only increases; therefore, we felt it necessary to mention it here so that competitors were prepared if they were to sign up for a live-judged show.

AFTER THE SHOW

Most competitors go into the show with a great plan; however, few have a plan in place for once the show wraps up. What you do at night after the show is dictated by your goal moving forward. If you are transitioning into the off-season, have an untracked meal out with the family and friends who came to your show to celebrate a successful contest season. As long as this meal does not become an all-out binge, you will be just fine. We cover the transition into the off-season in more detail in the next chapter.

However, if you plan to do another show within the next few weeks, you will not have as much leeway in terms of what you can do after your show. In fact, having a large untracked meal can significantly set you back in many cases. For example, if you came into your first show about two pounds (1 kg) over where you would ideally like to be, and your next show is in three weeks, eating a large untracked meal and gaining five pounds (2 kg) will make you look worse the next time you step onstage because it will require a faster ROL to be ready for the next show. But if you continue with your meal plan and keep aiming for your target ROL for the next three weeks, you will be at your best come show day. Do not let the meal after your show ruin your chances of success at shows the rest of your contest season. The food will still be there once you wrap up your last show of the year.

The stress and busyness of show day can cause it to go by all too quickly. Throughout the weekend, take multiple breaks to stop, look around, and appreciate all that you have accomplished to simply make it to the stage. You have worked hard for this, so make sure you soak it all in and enjoy it.

Take-Home Points

▶ You likely need to arrive at your show the day prior, when things like competitor check-in and drug testing occur. The day before the show will also be a great time to tie up any loose ends to ensure you are organized for show day.

▶ On show day, arrive early to the competition venue for the competitors meeting. Following the meeting, you have some time to prepare for prejudging where most judging occurs. You typically do routines and receive awards at the night show.

▶ Each show may do things a bit differently, so consult the schedule and information provided by the show promoter for more information.

▶ If you have another show in the next couple of weeks, bingeing the night after your show can affect how you look at the next show. The amount of leeway you have after your show depends on how much time you have until your next show and how much additional body fat you need to lose before then.

After the Event: Recovery and Recommendations

The show is over, the tan has faded, and you are back to your normal daily routine. Where do you go next?

Unsurprisingly, many competitors struggle with this. After you put so much effort into preparing for a competition, it can feel like a large void once the show is over. Often, there is also confusion as to what you should be doing during this time.

This chapter outlines how to handle the period after the show and the subsequent off-season to set yourself up for an improved physique the next time you step onstage.

POSTSHOW ANALYSIS

There is always a great deal of emotion surrounding a show. The process was long and grueling, and the show weekend was undoubtedly taxing and filled with emotional highs and lows. This leads many competitors to ignore a most important part of the postshow period, which is an analysis of what took place. Remember that each show you compete in is not only an accomplishment but also a learning experience. Successes and failures all serve as valuable learning tools.

After each show, make notes on what worked well and did not work well during your prep and what you did and did not do well along the way. For example, if you found a meal timing schedule that seemed to work well for you, note it. If you needed to get leaner, note it. If you realized training in the morning did not work well for you, make sure you note it. It is easy to say that you will remember these things later, but it is not as easy as you think to remember so many details.

Over the course of many shows, you can improve each prep. You can keep doing the things that work and change the things that do not. If you are purposeful about this, you will find ways to fine-tune the process. This analysis is one of those small things that turns average competitors into seasoned veterans.

COMPETING IN MULTIPLE SHOWS

We strongly recommend competing in multiple shows while stage-lean. Dieting for a show is extremely difficult and time-consuming. If you use the approaches we have outlined in this book, there will likely be a significant amount of time that you are not stage-lean between contest seasons. Doing multiple shows while stage-lean makes the most of the hard work you have put in during contest prep.

Many competitors attempt to do multiple competitions in a year by competing in the spring, again in the summer, and once again in the fall. Then they start right back again the following spring. However, this is not an optimal way to compete in multiple shows because it significantly increases the amount of time you are stage-lean, when hormone levels are less than ideal. It also limits the time you are able to spend out of a caloric deficit and above stage-lean levels of body fat. Ultimately, this cuts into progress long term.

Instead, we recommend competing in multiple competitions within a shorter time frame (usually around one to three months). This limits the time you need to stay stage-lean. It also maximizes the time spent in the off-season making progress while still allowing you to step onstage multiple times in a contest season.

As we noted in the previous chapter, those competing in multiple shows within a short time should not binge after the first competition because doing so adds unnecessary body fat. When you must diet off that regained body fat, you can lose additional muscle.

What you do between shows depends on your situation. If you still have more weight to lose heading into your next show, you need to hop back on your plan the day after your show and continue to shoot for loss. But if you were as lean as you needed to be for your first show, you need to start increasing intake and pulling back cardio to ensure you do not start dieting away muscle. You should aim for your current maintenance intake during this time since additional body fat loss is not necessary. Your current maintenance when stage-lean is lower than your maintenance at the start of prep.

PHYSIOLOGY OF BEING STAGE-LEAN

It is often said that being stage-lean looks awesome but feels terrible. This is due in part to the number of physiological changes that occur during contest prep. Before discussing what to do as you transition into the off-season, understand the state your body is in when you are stage-lean as you come out of your contest season. If you are drug-free and stage-lean, the following apply to you.

▶ *Reduced testosterone levels.* A 70 percent reduction (or more) in testosterone is observed in natural male bodybuilders during contest prep (6). Testosterone likely also decreases in females; however, since testosterone is lower initially, it does not have as large of an effect on muscle retention during contest prep. Interestingly, this may be one reason drug-free males anecdotally lose more muscle mass and strength during contest prep than drug-free females do. Regardless, significantly reduced testosterone levels have a detrimental effect on muscle size and strength gain. Fortunately, testosterone levels normalize once body fat is gained after a contest.

▶ *Menstrual cycle abnormalities.* Many women lose their menstrual cycles due to low caloric intake, high physical activity, extremely lean body composition, and abnormalities in hormone levels that occur during contest prep. Typically, normal menstrual cycles return once caloric intake and body fat begin to increase; however, it could take up to a year after a contest to regain a normal menstrual cycle (4). It may be unavoidable for a woman to lose her cycle to reach stage-lean levels of body fat. However, an effort should be made to have a normal menstrual cycle most of the time to avoid negative health consequences, such as bone loss and increased uterine cancer risk. This may mean a longer off-season is necessary for some women.

▶ *Reduced metabolic rate.* Metabolic rate is reduced during contest prep for several reasons, including decreased lean mass, decreased food intake, reduced nonexercise activity, decreased hormones, increased mitochondrial efficiency, and increased gut microbe extraction (5, 6, 8). For these reasons, plateaus in weight loss commonly occur during contest prep. The number of calories a person can consume to maintain weight will be reduced from the start of contest prep. However, metabolic rate also normalizes once caloric intake increases and body fat is gained.

▶ *Increased hunger.* Hormones that make you feel hungry (such as ghrelin) increase, while hormones that make you feel full (such as leptin) decrease during contest prep (6). Combine increased hunger with a reduced metabolic rate, and a competitor is set up for rapid weight regain. However, much like the other physiological changes discussed above, hunger hormones regulate when body fat percentage increases after a contest.

Remaining stage-lean in the long term can result in negative health consequences and significantly less physique progress since this physiological state is not conducive to muscle gain. If anything, you likely lose muscle over time due to low hormone levels. Therefore, you need to gain body fat after a competition to maximize progress during the off-season and in subsequent contest preps. And it will be important for your long-term health.

TRANSITIONING TO THE OFF-SEASON

An effective transition to the off-season requires attention the immediate few days after a show as well as the weeks or months until the next show. After a few untracked meals, bingeing should be avoided, and a competitor should look at an initial body fat regain and the overall off-season weight gain.

Bingeing

The worst way to handle the postshow period is to binge. If your final contest of the season is on a Saturday, we recommend enjoying some untracked food Saturday night and Sunday as long as it does not become an all-out binge. However, it is important to get back to some type of plan and consistency by Monday.

When Monday arrives, many people go back to what they were doing before starting contest prep. They either drastically increase caloric intake or just stop tracking intake altogether. At the same time, they drop cardio from several sessions weekly to none. Also, resistance training intensity and frequency may drop because they no longer have an immediate goal to train for.

The result of this approach is rapid weight and fat gain (2). In fact, a study of drug-free competitors found that most weight gained in the initial months after a contest is body fat (7). This means drug-free athletes are not "primed for muscle growth" as many believe and instead are primed for fat gain after a contest.

While fat gain is necessary following your show, rapid fat gain is not best for long-term progress. In some cases, weight gain may not stabilize until the person is at a higher body fat percentage than before starting contest prep. This is known as **body fat overshooting** (1).

After a competitor rapidly regains body fat, the first reaction is often to start dieting again. However, evidence from case studies of drug-free bodybuilders suggests that hormone levels and metabolic rate take time to normalize when body fat is regained after a contest (6). Moreover, there is some evidence that those who binge after a show do not see hormone normalization as quickly as those with more controlled weight gain (7). This means that if the person rapidly gains weight after the show and then immediately diets, he or she most likely requires a combination of lower calories and more cardio to reach a leaner body composition than what was needed during contest prep. Pushing caloric intake low and cardio high so quickly after a long contest prep period will likely only lower hormone levels and metabolic rate further. The result is an increased susceptibility to rapidly regaining body fat and increases the chance that you binge again. Avoid this cycle of bingeing and restricting.

If you have difficulty with bingeing postshow, we recommend that you consult with a qualified therapist who specializes in disordered eating patterns.

Initial Body Fat Regain

If you reached true stage-lean levels of body fat, you likely experienced several negative effects on hormone levels, energy, strength, muscle mass, metabolic rate, mood, and your relationship with food. Prolonging the amount of time in this state is not necessary: It may impact rate of progress in the off-season and may even be detrimental to long-term health.

The rate at which you aim to gain weight back after a competition depends on your situation. For example, if you struggled to stay consistent with your nutrition plan at the end of contest prep, pushing intake up faster and gaining a bit quicker may not be a bad idea. This allows you to find a middle ground where you can stay consistent and likely results in less rapid weight regain versus trying to follow an unsustainable plan and bingeing. On the other hand, if you did not truly get stage-lean and did not experience as many negative effects of being stage-lean, you may want to regain weight a bit slower since the amount of weight you will need to regain to feel more normal will be less. This would allow you to start your off-season (and hopefully your next contest prep) with a leaner body composition to help increase the chance you will be lean enough the next time you step onstage.

Pushing for quicker weight gain *initially* to add back body fat sooner may help normalize some of the negative effects of being stage-lean. However, do this in a controlled manner and not with an all-out binge. Once you are starting to feel more normal, slow the rate of gain to prevent excess body fat gain in the off-season so that you do not need to diet as soon or end up excessively above stage weight.

Some people struggle to see their contest body slowly disappearing as they add back body fat after the show. Although you need to regain body fat, in this case, gaining more slowly may be beneficial for motivation levels and psychological health. However, if you find that you are mentally struggling with postshow weight gain, reach out to a counselor specializing in disordered eating and body image.

Your target gain rate after the show ranges from 0.5 to 2 pounds (0.2-1 kg) weekly until you feel things are starting to normalize. For you, that point could be anywhere between 5 and 20 pounds (2-9 kg) over stage weight, depending on which division you competed in, how lean you were at your competition, your genetics, and other factors. This period can take one to three months and maybe more. However, we advise keeping a quicker rate of gain initially until you start to feel more normal, paying attention to factors such as your hunger, focus, energy, strength, sex drive, and sleep quality.

There is no single "best" way for everyone to increase intake initially after the show. In general, it is a good idea to initially increase your intake up to around (or just above) your current maintenance level, keeping in mind that your current maintenance is lower than your maintenance at the start of contest prep. Reduce cardio about 30 to 50 percent initially to help get you out of an energy deficit and around (or just above) your current maintenance.

From there, continue adjusting caloric intake up and cardio down to maintain your target rate of gain in the initial weeks postshow until you have gained enough body fat that you start to feel more normal again. If you are not gaining weight coming out of a show, larger increases may be necessary to make sure you start gaining sooner rather than later to avoid staying stage-lean long-term.

Off-Season Weight Gain

After you reach a more sustainable body composition, where hormones, strength, metabolic rate, and your overall feeling of "normal" start to return, you need to slow your rate of gain to prevent excessive fat gain and allow yourself to stay out of a deficit for a prolonged period. A larger caloric surplus and faster rate of gain will not result in more muscle gain. It only results in more body fat gain (3). For this reason, after an initial gain, we recommend the monthly gain rate slow to one pound (0.5 kg) at the most or two pounds (0.9 kg) for younger competitors newer to the sport. Drug-free females may even want to aim for a slower gain per month.

Where you allow your weight to drift in the off-season depends on many factors. As with most things in this sport, it is not one-size-fits-all. Most people have a range of weight where they can sit comfortably. Going below this range takes restraint and may result in detrimental effects to hormones and other body processes, as previously discussed. On the other hand, venturing above this range often requires force-feeding and results in excessive fat gain (thereby leading to a more difficult prep the next time). An ideal amount of gain for a competitor allows him or her to sit somewhere within this comfortable weight range during the off-season.

FAQ: Does everyone need to regain body fat after a show?

For most competitors, weight gain after the contest will be necessary. If you truly got stage-lean, you need to gain weight after the show (discussed in detail previously). Your plan should include a quick increase in intake and decrease in cardio to allow you to gain and return to a more sustainable body fat percentage.

However, someone who does not get stage-lean may not need to gain a lot of weight. As we mentioned earlier, if you are not ready for a show, our recommendation would be to pick a later show to give yourself more time. But if that is not possible and you step onstage with at least 10 to 15 pounds (4-7 kg) to lose, you may still be at a body fat percentage that is healthy and sustainable (or at least not far away from it). This means the amount of weight you need to gain back is less than the competitor who did get stage-lean.

One common mistake competitors make is not getting stage-lean but still treating the postshow period as if they had. This results in unnecessary weight gain and increases the chances they will not get stage-lean the next time around.

Competitors who have been stage-lean know that when they get close to stage-lean, the amount of time thinking about food significantly increases. Meals become much more elaborate and time-intensive, and a person may try to milk everything he or she can out of a limited intake. This relationship with food is not necessarily normal, and there should be an effort in the off-season to establish a healthier relationship with food, where you are not as food-focused. Allowing body weight and body fat to come up to a level that results in you not being food-focused is important for long-term psychological health.

In addition, younger competitors who have not been training as long have a greater capacity for growth because their hormone levels are closer to optimal, and they are further from their genetic ceiling. Often, they also have a faster metabolic rate, which makes dieting down for shows easier. As a result, a younger competitor can let his or her weight drift up a bit more to take advantage of a prime growing period, while an older competitor may be better staying a bit closer to stage weight.

Males have a greater capacity for muscle growth than females do because of higher levels of anabolic hormones such as testosterone. In addition, males tend to have a higher metabolic rate due to higher body mass and muscle mass. Therefore, a female competitor may want to stay a bit closer to stage-lean than her male counterpart does.

Consider your level of conditioning at your last competition, the length of your off-season, and how easily you get stage-lean when you are determining what your weight should be. People who still had a good amount of weight to lose at their last show need to gain less weight in the off-season than competitors with striations in their glutes and veins in their hamstrings do. The division you compete in may play a role as well, because conditioning does not have to be as high in bikini as in bodybuilding. This means that a bikini competitor will typically not have to gain as much weight in the off-season as a bodybuilder does, even if both reached the conditioning standards of their division at their competition. If your off-season is short or you have difficulty losing weight, it may be advisable to stay a bit closer to stage weight.

A primary goal of an off-season is to add muscle and improve your physique before your next competition. Staying stage-lean, or close to it, will result in strength levels remaining low, thereby reducing the amount of muscle mass you can gain. In general, it is a good idea to let weight increase to a point where strength is high to maximize progress. However, you will reach diminished returns, where you are not seeing additional strength gain for the weight you are adding. This is a signal that you should not allow your weight to increase further above stage weight in the off-season.

It is also important to address the psychological effects of weight regain. Psychological disorders are common among physique competitors and should be addressed with a professional before dieting down for a competition. Dieting down for a show will usually only amplify preexisting issues with food, exercise, and body image. Even in competitors without signs of preexisting psychological disorders, contest prep may bring some of these issues to the surface. As a result, some people may struggle more with weight gain after a show than others do. This does not mean that they should stay stage-lean, but they may want to slow the rate at which they regain weight or stay a bit closer to stage-lean, provided that they gain enough to normalize things hormonally and metabolically. If you struggle with weight gain after the contest, we recommend consulting a professional to work through things before jumping back into contest prep.

As you may expect, there is no off-season weight gain amount ideal for everyone. Optimal off-season weight gain depends on the factors we discussed. Some competitors may only need to regain 5 to 10 pounds (2-5 kg), while others may be best off gaining more than 30 pounds (more than 14 kg) during their off-season.

You should aim to gain enough weight back that you feel normal and are gaining strength at a weight you can hold without feeling restricted about food. However, you also want to not get excessively far over stage-lean to avoid having to lose an excessive amount of body fat during your next contest prep. While you can always run a short cut, typically referred to as a **mini cut**, to lean out a bit in the off-season, the most time should be spent both at a sustainable body fat percentage and out of a deficit during your off-season without getting excessively far over stage weight.

Each time you diet down for a contest season, your goal should be to look better than the previous contest season. While most people put a greater amount of effort and focus into their contest prep, that is not the time you will make most of your improvements. Once you have mastered the art of the contest prep, you make true progress in the off-season. So, give this special time the attention, focus, and effort it truly deserves.

Take-Home Points

▶ Assess your physique following your competition to ensure you create an off-season plan that results in an improved physique the next time you step onstage.

▶ If you do multiple shows within the same contest season, do them over a one- to three-month period. Be consistent with your nutrition plan postshow and do not binge, especially if you have another show within a few weeks.

▶ If you struggle in any way with bingeing or body image associated with weight regain following a competition, we encourage you to reach out to a counselor specialized in body image and disordered eating patterns.

▶ Many factors affect how quickly you gain weight postshow and how high you allow your weight to drift in the off-season. However, if you reached stage-lean levels of body fat, you need to gain weight back after your show.

▶ There is no amount of off-season weight gain that is ideal for everyone!

EPILOGUE

Competitive bodybuilding is an incredibly difficult sport that few people have the dedication to endure. While many people take diet and training seriously, few have the mental and physical fortitude to tackle what is required to get on stage. Athletes in other sports train hard and then go home to mentally and physically relax, but competitive bodybuilders must remain dedicated throughout every resistance training and cardio session, each meal, and every night when they are having difficulty falling asleep because they are hungry. There is no reprieve from the demands of such a life. Our minds and bodies are called to remember our task nearly every moment.

When most of us enter the sport, we do so with only dreams of what we will look like one day. We visualize chiseled abs, mountainous biceps, and capped delts that we will be proud of. In our zeal to achieve this ideal body we want so much, we resolve to do "whatever it takes" to get where we aim to be. This mindset has built many champions over the years. However, this mentality has also led many athletes, not just bodybuilders, to their ultimate failure.

The problem with doing whatever it takes to win is that many people often do not take the time to identify what is required to accomplish that. Blind hard work is never the answer. In bodybuilding, that mindset is often applauded, even when people are completely off base. Yet, blind hard work will not put them any closer to their goals. If a marathon runner were to run 35 miles in the wrong direction rather than the required 26.2 miles on a race course, he or she would have worked harder (ran farther) than fellow racers yet lost the race. Put forth significant effort but always assess if the effort is necessary, useful, and specific to your goal.

Even after we remove all unnecessary, useless, or vague effort, what we are left with in the bodybuilding journey is simply difficult beyond measure. In this sport, we must demand more of ourselves than anyone else would ever demand from us and expect more of ourselves than others would ever expect from us. The fastest route to mediocrity is to only meet the standards that others set for us. The grueling nature of bodybuilding itself, particularly contest prep, tends to attract those who want to test themselves against the challenge and achieve a body that *others simply cannot*.

In this sport, we derive joy from our results. Who among us does not delight in looking in the mirror and seeing the fruits of our labor or experiencing the feeling of winning a big show? It feels good to work for something and then see it pay off. However, what will keep you going when progress slows down (and it will), when you have a bad placing at a show (and you will), or when the timetable to reach your goals seems like it will take *years* rather than weeks (because it does)? Do you have it in you to keep going? For many, the answer is no.

Bodybuilders tend to look to the future with rose-colored glasses. They project forward and think, "I'll be happier when I'm bigger and leaner." Or, "I'll be happy when I win that show." This attitude places the entirety of one's happiness on the *result*. This leads to an almost desperate mentality to get results in which every ounce of short-term progress takes on momentous importance.

Ironically, to achieve happiness through results and achievement, the process usually becomes a source of despair and desperation. Once that sets in, each personal record in the gym and each show placing is viewed as a live-or-die situation. The problem is that in bodybuilding, you lose *far* more shows than you win, and beyond the first five years of training, personal records in the gym will become rare. Adopting a live-or-die mentality means that you die over and over.

Rather than living and dying with every success and failure, learn to enjoy the successes, learn from the failures, and move on. Success and failure are only temporary states. *Each success only lasts until our next failure, and each failure only lasts until our next success.* For this reason, we should not get caught up in any single instance of either type. We enjoy, we learn, and we move on.

This arduous process makes bodybuilding so intolerable and yet so beautiful. Competitors who get to the competitive arena often only last about three to four years before they eventually quit. It wears on them so greatly that they cannot sustain the process long. The sad part is that achieving one's personal best in bodybuilding takes longer than just a few years; it usually takes a decade or more. So what separates those who can last from those who cannot? What is that secret ingredient that allows some to endure while others flame out?

The answer to these questions is simple. The key to enduring all the hardships in this sport over the long haul is enjoyment. The *result* of the bodybuilding process cannot and must not be the only source of our joy. *We must learn to derive joy from the process itself if we wish to last.* True happiness does not come from any single thing, even bodybuilding results; it comes from having an abundance of sources of joy in our lives. Bodybuilding must add to life's total joy. If it does not do that, then we cannot be expected to have the will to continue doing it.

If everything you do in this sport is viewed as something to "simply endure" to reach an end goal that will be your only source of joy, you will be miserable. *Successful people do not live through sacrifice. They live through passion.* You must love what you do, not just the result of what you do. There is a clear difference between the person who continues for two decades and the person who continues for only two years. The former will wake up most days for two decades and be excited for what he or she gets to do that day, but the latter will wake up every day for two years excited for what he or she hopes to accomplish someday, yet dreads what must be done to get it.

In the end, bodybuilding can be an incredibly powerful positive force in the lives of those who take up the challenge. It tests us our will, teaches us our power, and has the ability to make us better, both mentally and physically. The reasons we started in this sport are rarely the reasons we stay. The improvements we make are rarely what we envisioned at the outset, but they are a source of more pride than we ever could have imagined. As you progress along your journey, you must work hard, test your limits, and give every ounce of energy to achieve your full potential. Always remember, though, to enjoy the privilege, benefits, and beauty that this sport has to offer, because they are plentiful.

REFERENCES

CHAPTER 1

1. Bamman, MM, Hunter, GR, Newton, LE, Roney, RK, and Khaled, MA. Changes in body composition, diet, and strength of body-builders during the 12 weeks prior to competition. *J Sports Med Phys Fitness* 33:383-391, 1993.

2. Helms, ER, Aragon, AA, and Fitschen, PJ. Evidence-based recommendations for natural bodybuilding contest preparation: nutrition and supplementation. *J Int Soc Sports Nutr* 11:20, 2014.

3. Helms, ER, Fitschen, PJ, Aragon, AA, Cronin, J, and Schoenfeld, BJ. Recommendations for natural bodybuilding contest preparation: resistance and cardiovascular training. *J Sports Med Phys Fitness* 55:164-178, 2015.

4. Kleiner, SM, Bazzarre, TL, and Litchford, MD. Metabolic profiles, diet, and health practices of championship male and female bodybuilders. *J Am Diet Assoc* 90:962-967, 1990.

5. Steen, SN. Precontest strategies of a male bodybuilder. *Int J Sport Nutr* 1:69-78, 1991.

6. Trexler, ET, Hirsch, KR, Campbell, BI, and Smith-Ryan, AE. Physiological changes following competition in male and female physique athletes: a pilot study. *Int J Sport Nutr Exerc Metab* 27:458-466, 2017.

7. van der Ploeg, GE, Brooks, AG, Withers, RT, Dollman, J, Leaney, F, and Chatterton, BE. Body composition changes in female bodybuilders during preparation for competition. *Eur J Clin Nutr* 55:268-277, 2001.

CHAPTER 4

1. Hubal, MJ, Gordish-Dressman, H, Thompson, PD, Price, TB, Hoffman, EP, Angelopoulos, TJ, Gordon, PM, Moyna, NM, Pescatello, LS, Visich, PS, Zoeller, RF, Seip, RL, and Clarkson, PM. Variability in muscle size and strength gain after unilateral resistance training. *Med Sci Sports Exerc* 37:964-972, 2005.

2. Pardue, A, Trexler, ET, and Sprod, LK. Case study: unfavorable but transient physiological changes during contest preparation in a drug-free male bodybuilder. *Int J Sport Nutr Exerc Metab* 27:550-559, 2017.

3. Rossow, LM, Fukuda, DH, Fahs, CA, Loenneke, JP, and Stout, JR. Natural bodybuilding competition preparation and recovery: a 12-month case study. *Int J Sports Physiol Perform* 8:582-592, 2013.

CHAPTER 5

1. Azizi, F. Effect of dietary composition on fasting-induced changes in serum thyroid hormones and thyrotropin. *Metabolism* 27:935-942, 1978.

2. Bhasin, S, Storer, TW, Berman, N, Callegari, C, Clevenger, B,

Phillips, J, Bunnell, TJ, Tricker, R, Shirazi, A, and Casaburi, R. The effects of supraphysiologic doses of testosterone on muscle size and strength in normal men. *N Engl J Med* 335:1-7, 1996.

3. Burke, LM, Loucks, AB, and Broad, N. Energy and carbohydrate for training and recovery. *J Sports Sci* 24:675-685, 2006.

4. Byrne, NM, Sainsbury, A, King, NA, Hills, AP, and Wood, RE. Intermittent energy restriction improves weight loss efficiency in obese men: the MATADOR study. *Int J Obes (Lond)* 42:129-138, 2018.

5. Chaston, TB, Dixon, JB, and O'Brien, PE. Changes in fat-free mass during significant weight loss: a systematic review. *Int J Obes (Lond)* 31:743-750, 2007.

6. Garthe, I, Raastad, T, Refsnes, PE, Koivisto, A, and Sundgot-Borgen, J. Effect of two different weight-loss rates on body composition and strength and power-related performance in elite athletes. *Int J Sport Nutr Exerc Metab* 21:97-104, 2011.

7. Halliday, TM, Loenneke, JP, and Davy, BM. Dietary intake, body composition, and menstrual cycle changes during competition preparation and recovery in a drug-free figure competitor: a case study. *Nutrients* 8:740, 2016.

8. Helms, ER, Aragon, AA, and Fitschen, PJ. Evidence-based recommendations for natural bodybuilding contest preparation: nutrition and supplementation. *J Int Soc Sports Nutr* 11:20, 2014.

9. Kistler, BM, Fitschen, PJ, Ranadive, SM, Fernhall, B, and Wilund, KR. Case study: natural bodybuilding contest preparation. *Int J Sport Nutr Exerc Metab* 24:694-700, 2014.

10. Knuth, ND, Johannsen, DL, Tamboli, RA, Marks-Shulman, PA, Huizenga, R, Chen, KY, Abumrad, NN, Ravussin, E, and Hall, KD. Metabolic adaptation following massive weight loss is related to the degree of energy imbalance and changes in circulating leptin. *Obesity (Silver Spring)* 22:2563-2569, 2014.

11. Kreitzman, SN, Coxon, AY, and Szaz, KF. Glycogen storage: illusions of easy weight loss, excessive weight regain, and distortions in estimates of body composition. *Am J Clin Nutr* 56:292S-293S, 1992.

12. Robinson, SL, Lambeth-Mansell, A, Gillibrand, G, Smith-Ryan, A, and Bannock, L. A nutrition and conditioning intervention for natural bodybuilding contest preparation: case study. *J Int Soc Sports Nutr* 12:20, 2015.

13. Rodriguez, NR, DiMarco, NM, and Langley, S. American College of Sports Medicine position stand. Nutrition and athletic performance. *Med Sci Sports Exerc* 41:709-731, 2009.

14. Romon, M, Lebel, P, Velly, C, Marecaux, N, Fruchart, JC, and Dallongeville, J. Leptin response to carbohydrate or fat meal and association with subsequent satiety and energy intake. *Am J Physiol* 277:E855-861, 1999.

15. Rossow, LM, Fukuda, DH, Fahs, CA, Loenneke, JP, and Stout, JR. Natural bodybuilding competition preparation and recovery: a 12-month case study. *Int J Sports Physiol Perform* 8:582-592, 2013.

16. Trexler, ET, Hirsch, KR, Campbell, BI, and Smith-Ryan, AE. Physiological changes following competition in male and female physique athletes: a pilot study. *Int J Sport Nutr Exerc Metab* 27:458-466, 2017.

17. Trexler, ET, Smith-Ryan, AE, and Norton, LE. Metabolic adaptation to weight loss: implications for the athlete. *J Int Soc Sports Nutr* 11:7, 2014.

18. Wing, RR and Jeffery, RW. Prescribed "breaks" as a means to disrupt weight control efforts. *Obes Res* 11:287-291, 2003.

CHAPTER 6

1. Abargouei, AS, Janghorbani, M, Salehi-Marzijarani, M, and Esmaillzadeh, A. Effect of dairy consumption on weight and body composition in adults: a systematic review and meta-analysis of randomized controlled clinical trials. *Int J Obes (Lond)* 36:1485-1493, 2012.

2. Anderson, JW, Baird, P, Davis, RH, Jr., Ferreri, S, Knudtson, M, Koraym, A, Waters, V, and Williams, CL. Health benefits of dietary fiber. *Nutr Rev* 67:188-205, 2009.

3. Antonio, J and Ellerbroek, A. Case reports on well-trained bodybuilders: two years on a high-protein diet. *J Ex Physiol* 21:14-24, 2018.

4. Antonio, J, Ellerbroek, A, Silver, T, Vargas, L, Tamayo, A, Buehn, R, and Peacock, C. A high-protein diet has no harmful effects: a one-year crossover study in resistance-trained males *J Nutr Metab* 2016. [e-pub ahead of print].

5. Azizi, F. Effect of dietary composition on fasting-induced changes in serum thyroid hormones and thyrotropin. *Metabolism* 27:935-942, 1978.

6. Bandegan, A, Courtney-Martin, G, Rafii, M, Pencharz, PB, and Lemon, PW. Indicator amino acid-derived estimate of dietary protein requirement for male bodybuilders on a nontraining day is several-fold greater than the current recommended dietary allowance. *J Nutr* 147:850-857, 2017.

7. Bantle, JP, Raatz, SK, Thomas, W, and Georgopoulos, A. Effects of dietary fructose on plasma lipids in healthy subjects. *Am J Clin Nutr* 72:1128-1134, 2000.

8. Bohe, J, Low, JF, Wolfe, RR, and Rennie, MJ. Latency and duration of stimulation of human muscle protein synthesis during continuous infusion of amino acids. *J Physiol* 532:575-579, 2001.

9. Bray, GA, Most, M, Rood, J, Redmann, S, and Smith, SR. Hormonal responses to a fast-food meal compared with nutritionally comparable meals of different composition. *Ann Nutr Metab* 51:163-171, 2007.

10. Byrne, NM, Sainsbury, A, King, NA, Hills, AP, and Wood, RE. Intermittent energy restriction improves weight loss efficiency in obese men: the MATADOR study. *Int J Obes (Lond)* 42:129-138, 2018.

11. Cameron, JD, Cyr, MJ, and Doucet, E. Increased meal frequency does not promote greater weight loss in subjects who were prescribed an 8-week equi-energetic energy-restricted diet. *Br J Nutr* 103:1098-1101, 2010.

12. Campbell, BI, Aguilar, D, Conlin, L, Vargas, A, Schoenfeld, BJ, Corson, A, Gai, C, Best, S, Galvan, E, and Couvillion, K. Effects of high vs. low protein intake on body composition and maximal strength in aspiring female physique athletes engaging in an 8-week resistance training program. *Int J Sport Nutr Exerc Metab* 1-21, 2018.

13. Champagne, CM, Bray, GA, Kurtz, AA, Monteiro, JB, Tucker, E, Volaufova, J, and Delany, JP. Energy intake and energy expenditure: a controlled study comparing dietitians and non-dietitians. *J Am Diet Assoc* 102:1428-1432, 2002.

14. de Souza, RJ, Mente, A, Maroleanu, A, Cozma, AI, Ha, V, Kishibe, T, Uleryk, E, Budylowski, P, Schunemann, H, Beyene, J, and Anand, SS. Intake of saturated and trans unsaturated fatty acids and risk of all cause mortality, cardiovascular disease, and type 2 diabetes: systematic review and meta-analysis of observational studies. *BMJ* 351:h3978, 2015.

15. Ferraro, R, Lillioja, S, Fontvieille, AM, Rising, R, Bogardus, C, and Ravussin, E. Lower sedentary metabolic rate in women compared with men. *J Clin Invest* 90:780-784, 1992.

16. Haff, GG, Stone, MH, Warren, BJ, Keith, R, Johnson, RL, Nieman, DC, Williams, F, and Kirksey, KB. The effect of carbohydrate supplementation on multiple sessions and bouts of resistance exercise. *J Strength Cond Res* 13:111-117, 1999.

17. Haff, GG, Stone, MH, Warren, BJ, Keith, R, Johnson, RL, Nieman, DC, Williams, F, and Kirksey, KB. The effect of carbohydrate supplementation on multiple sessions and bouts of resistance exercise. *J Strength Cond Res* 13:111-117, 1999.

18. Haffner, SM, D'Agostino, R, Saad, MF, Rewers, M, Mykkanen, L, Selby, J, Howard, G, Savage, PJ, Hamman, RF, Wegenknecht, LE, and Bergman, RN. Increased insulin resistance and insulin secretion in nondiabetic African Americans and Hispanics compared with non-Hispanic whites: the insulin resistance atherosclerosis atudy. *Diabetes* 45:742-748, 1996.

19. Halliday, TM, Loenneke, JP, and Davy, BM. Dietary intake, body composition, and menstrual cycle changes during competition preparation and recovery in a drug-free figure competitor: a case study. *Nutrients* 8:740, 2016.

20. Hammad, S, Pu, S, and Jones, PJ. Current evidence supporting the link between dietary fatty acids and cardiovascular disease. *Lipids* 51:507-517, 2016.

21. Helms, ER, Aragon, AA, and Fitschen, PJ. Evidence-based recommendations for natural bodybuilding contest preparation: nutrition and supplementation. *J Int Soc Sports Nutr* 11:20, 2014.

22. Hickson, JF, Jr., Johnson, TE, Lee, W, and Sidor, RJ. Nutrition and the precontest preparations of a male bodybuilder. *J Am Diet Assoc* 90:264-267, 1990.

23. Jeukendrup, AE, Wagenmakers, AJ, Stegen, JH, Gijsen, AP, Brouns, F, and Saris, WH. Carbohydrate ingestion can completely suppress endogenous glucose production during exercise. *Am J Physiol* 276:E672-E683, 1999.

24. Kistler, BM, Fitschen, PJ, Ranadive, SM, Fernhall, B, and Wilund, KR. Case study: natural bodybuilding contest preparation. *Int J Sport Nutr Exerc Metab* 24:694-700, 2014.

25. Kleiner, SM, Bazzarre, TL, and Litchford, MD. Metabolic profiles, diet, and health practices of championship male and female bodybuilders. *J Am Diet Assoc* 90:962-967, 1990.

26. Lamar-Hildebrand, N, Saldanha, L, and Endres, J. Dietary and exercise practices of college-aged female bodybuilders. *J Am Diet Assoc* 89:1308-1310, 1989.

27. Leaf, A and Antonio, J. The effects of overfeeding on body composition: the role of macronutrient composition: a narrative review. *Int J Exerc Sci* 10:1275-1296, 2017.

28. Lichtman, SW, Pisarska, K, Berman, ER, Pestone, M, Dowling, H, Offenbacher, E, Weisel, H, Heshka, S, Matthews, DE, and Heymsfield, SB. Discrepancy between self-reported and actual caloric

intake and exercise in obese subjects. *N Engl J Med* 327:1893-1898, 1992.

29. Macdiarmid, J and Blundell, J. Assessing dietary intake: who, what and why of under-reporting. *Nutr Res Rev* 11:231-253, 1998.

30. Maclean, PS, Bergouignan, A, Cornier, MA, and Jackman, MR. Biology's response to dieting: the impetus for weight regain. *Am J Physiol Regul Integr Comp Physiol* 301:R581-600, 2011.

31. Magnuson, BA, Burdock, GA, Doull, J, Kroes, RM, Marsh, GM, Pariza, MW, Spencer, PS, Waddell, WJ, Walker, R, and Williams, GM. Aspartame: a safety evaluation based on current use levels, regulations, and toxicological and epidemiological studies. *Crit Rev Toxicol* 37:629-727, 2007.

32. Mozaffarian, D, Micha, R, and Wallace, S. Effects on coronary heart disease of increasing polyunsaturated fat in place of saturated fat: a systematic review and meta-analysis of randomized controlled trials. *PLoS Med* 7:e1000252, 2010.

33. Phillips, SM. A brief review of critical processes in exercise-induced muscular hypertrophy. *Sports Med* 44 Suppl 1:S71-77, 2014.

34. Res, PT, Groen, B, Pennings, B, Beelen, M, Wallis, GA, Gijsen, AP, Senden, JM, and LJ, VANL. Protein ingestion before sleep improves postexercise overnight recovery. *Med Sci Sports Exerc* 44:1560-1569, 2012.

35. Robergs, RA, Pearson, DR, Costill, DL, Fink, WJ, Pascoe, DD, Benedict, MA, Lambert, CP, and Zachweija, JJ. Muscle glycogenolysis during differing intensities of weight-resistance exercise. *J Appl Physiol (1985)* 70:1700-1706, 1991.

36. Robinson, SL, Lambeth-Mansell, A, Gillibrand, G, Smith-Ryan, A, and Bannock, L. A nutrition and conditioning intervention for natural bodybuilding contest preparation: case study. *J Int Soc Sports Nutr* 12:20, 2015.

37. Rogers, PJ, Hogenkamp, PS, de Graaf, C, Higgs, S, Lluch, A, Ness, AR, Penfold, C, Perry, R, Putz, P, Yeomans, MR, and Mela, DJ. Does low-energy sweetener consumption affect energy intake and body weight? A systematic review, including meta-analyses, of the evidence from human and animal studies. *Int J Obes (Lond)* 40:381-394, 2016.

38. Romon, M, Lebel, P, Velly, C, Marecaux, N, Fruchart, JC, and Dallongeville, J. Leptin response to carbohydrate or fat meal and association with subsequent satiety and energy intake. *Am J Physiol* 277:E855-861, 1999.

39. Rossow, LM, Fukuda, DH, Fahs, CA, Loenneke, JP, and Stout, JR. Natural bodybuilding competition preparation and recovery: a 12-month case study. *Int J Sports Physiol Perform* 8:582-592, 2013.

40. Sandoval, WM, Heyward, VH, and Lyons, TM. Comparison of body composition, exercise and nutritional profiles of female and male body builders at competition. *J Sports Med Phys Fitness* 29:63-70, 1989.

41. Schoenfeld, BJ, Aragon, AA, and Krieger, JW. The effect of protein timing on muscle strength and hypertrophy: a meta-analysis. *J Int Soc Sports Nutr* 10:53, 2013.

42. Seimon, RV, Roekenes, JA, Zibellini, J, Zhu, B, Gibson, AA, Hills, AP, Wood, RE, King, NA, Byrne, NM, and Sainsbury, A. Do intermittent diets provide physiological benefits over continuous diets for weight loss? A systematic review of clinical trials. *Mol Cell Endocrinol* 418 Pt 2:153-172, 2015.

43. Siri-Tarino, PW, Sun, Q, Hu, FB, and Krauss, RM. Meta-analysis of prospective cohort studies evaluating the association of saturated fat with cardiovascular disease. *Am J Clin Nutr* 91:535-546, 2010.

44. Smith, CF, Williamson, DA, Bray, GA, and Ryan, DH. Flexible vs. rigid dieting strategies: relationship with adverse behavioral outcomes. *Appetite* 32:295-305, 1999.

45. Sofer, S, Eliraz, A, Kaplan, S, Voet, H, Fink, G, Kima, T, and Madar, Z. Greater weight loss and hormonal changes after 6 months diet with carbohydrates eaten mostly at dinner. *Obesity (Silver Spring)* 19:2006-2014, 2011.

46. Spaeth, AM, Dinges, DF, and Goel, N. Resting metabolic rate varies by race and by sleep duration. *Obesity (Silver Spring)* 23:2349-2356, 2015.

47. Steen, SN. Precontest strategies of a male bodybuilder. *Int J Sport Nutr* 1:69-78, 1991.

48. Thomas, DM, Martin, CK, Lettieri, S, Bredlau, C, Kaiser, K, Church, T, Bouchard, C, and Heymsfield, SB. Can a weight loss of one pound a week be achieved with a 3,500-kcal deficit? Commentary on a commonly accepted rule. *Int J Obes (Lond)* 37:1611-1613, 2013.

49. Trexler, ET, Smith-Ryan, AE, and Norton, LE. Metabolic adaptation to weight loss: implications for the athlete. *J Int Soc Sports Nutr* 11:7, 2014.

50. van Marken Lichtenbelt, WD, Hartgens, F, Vollaard, NB, Ebbing, S, and Kuipers, H. Body composition changes in bodybuilders: a method comparison. *Med Sci Sports Exerc* 36:490-497, 2004.

51. Varady, KA. Intermittent versus daily calorie restriction: which diet regimen is more effective for weight loss? *Obes Rev* 12:e593-e601, 2011.

52. Weigle, DS, Breen, PA, Matthys, CC, Callahan, HS, Meeuws, KE, Burden, VR, and Purnell, JQ. A high-protein diet induces sustained reductions in appetite, ad libitum caloric intake, and body weight despite compensatory changes in diurnal plasma leptin and ghrelin concentrations. *Am J Clin Nutr* 82:41-48, 2005.

53. Wing, RR and Jeffery, RW. Prescribed "breaks" as a means to disrupt weight control efforts. *Obes Res* 11:287-291, 2003.

CHAPTER 7

1. Amirthalingam, T, Mavros, Y, Wilson, GC, Clarke, JL, Mitchell, L, and Hackett, DA. Effects of a modified German volume training program on muscular hypertrophy and strength. *J Strength Cond Res* 31:3109-3119, 2017.

2. Bartholomew, JB, Stults-Kolehmainen, MA, Elrod, CC, and Todd, JS. Strength gains after resistance training: the effect of stressful, negative life events. *J Strength Cond Res* 22:1215-1221, 2008.

3. Bravata, DM, Smith-Spangler, C, Sundaram, V, Gienger, AL, Lin, N, Lewis, R, Stave, CD, Olkin, I, and Sirard, JR. Using pedometers to increase physical activity and improve health: a systematic review. *JAMA* 298:2296-2304, 2007.

4. Campos, GE, Luecke, TJ, Wendeln, HK, Toma, K, Hagerman, FC, Murray, TF, Ragg, KE, Ratamess, NA, Kraemer, WJ, and Staron, RS. Muscular adaptations in response to three different resistance-training regimens: specificity of repetition maximum training zones. *Eur J Appl Physiol* 88:50-60, 2002.

5. Coffey, VG and Hawley, JA. Concurrent exercise training: do opposites distract? *J Physiol* 595:2883-2896, 2016.

6. Davies, T, Orr, R, Halaki, M, and Hackett, D. Effect of training

leading to repetition failure on muscular strength: a systematic review and meta-analysis. *Sports Med* 46:487-502, 2015.

7. de Lacerda, LT, Costa, HCM, Diniz, RCR, Lima, FV, Andrade, AGP, Tourino, FD, Bemben, MG, and Chagas, MH. Variations in repetition duration and repetition numbers influences muscular activation and blood lactate response in protocols equalized by time under tension. *J Strength Cond Res*, 2015. [e-pub ahead of print].

8. Fonseca, RM, Roschel, H, Tricoli, V, de Souza, EO, Wilson, JM, Laurentino, GC, Aihara, AY, de Souza Leao, AR, and Ugrinowitsch, C. Changes in exercises are more effective than in loading schemes to improve muscle strength. *J Strength Cond Res* 28:3085-3092, 2014.

9. Fry, AC and Kraemer, WJ. Resistance exercise overtraining and overreaching. Neuroendocrine responses. *Sports Med* 23:106-129, 1997.

10. Headley, SA, Henry, K, Nindl, BC, Thompson, BA, Kraemer, WJ, and Jones, MT. Effects of lifting tempo on one repetition maximum and hormonal responses to a bench press protocol. *J Strength Cond Res* 25:406-413, 2011.

11. Henselmans, M and Schoenfeld, BJ. The effect of inter-set rest intervals on resistance exercise-induced muscle hypertrophy. *Sports Med* 44:1635-1643, 2014.

12. Kim, E, Dear, A, Ferguson, SL, Seo, D, and Bemben, MG. Effects of 4 weeks of traditional resistance training vs. superslow strength training on early phase adaptations in strength, flexibility, and aerobic capacity in college-aged women. *J Strength Cond Res* 25:3006-3013, 2011.

13. King, NA, Caudwell, P, Hopkins, M, Byrne, NM, Colley, R, Hills, AP, Stubbs, JR, and Blundell, JE. Metabolic and behavioral compensatory responses to exercise interventions: barriers to weight loss. *Obesity (Silver Spring)* 15:1373-1383, 2007.

14. Klemp, A, Dolan, C, Quiles, JM, Blanco, R, Zoeller, RF, Graves, BS, and Zourdos, MC. Volume-equated high- and low-repetition daily undulating programming strategies produce similar hypertrophy and strength adaptations. *Appl Physiol Nutr Metab* 41:699-705, 2016.

15. Krieger, JW. Single vs. multiple sets of resistance exercise for muscle hypertrophy: a meta-analysis. *J Strength Cond Res* 24:1150-1159, 2010.

16. Larsson, ME, Kall, I, and Nilsson-Helander, K. Treatment of patellar tendinopathy: a systematic review of randomized controlled trials. *Knee Surg Sports Traumatol Arthrosc* 20:1632-1646, 2012.

17. Levine, JA. Nonexercise activity thermogenesis: liberating the life-force. *J Intern Med* 262:273-287, 2007.

18. Maclean, PS, Bergouignan, A, Cornier, MA, and Jackman, MR. Biology's response to dieting: the impetus for weight regain. *Am J Physiol Regul Integr Comp Physiol* 301:R581-600, 2011.

19. McMahon, GE, Morse, CI, Burden, A, Winwood, K, and Onambele, GL. Impact of range of motion during ecologically valid resistance training protocols on muscle size, subcutaneous fat, and strength. *J Strength Cond Res* 28:245-255, 2014.

20. Melanson, EL, Sharp, TA, Seagle, HM, Horton, TJ, Donahoo, WT, Grunwald, GK, Hamilton, JT, and Hill, JO. Effect of exercise intensity on 24-h energy expenditure and nutrient oxidation. *J Appl Physiol (1985)* 92:1045-1052, 2002.

21. Miller, BF, Olesen, JL, Hansen, M, Dossing, S, Crameri, RM, Welling, RJ, Langberg, H, Flyvbjerg, A, Kjaer, M, Babraj, JA, Smith, K, and Rennie, MJ. Coordinated collagen and muscle protein synthesis in human patella tendon and quadriceps muscle

after exercise. *J Physiol* 567:1021-1033, 2005.

22. Morton, RW, Oikawa, SY, Wavell, CG, Mazara, N, McGlory, C, Quadrilatero, J, Baechler, BL, Baker, SK, and Phillips, SM. Neither load nor systemic hormones determine resistance training-mediated hypertrophy or strength gains in resistance-trained young men. *J Appl Physiol (1985)* 121:129-138, 2016.

23. Phillips, SM, Tipton, KD, Aarsland, A, Wolf, SE, and Wolfe, RR. Mixed muscle protein synthesis and breakdown after resistance exercise in humans. *Am J Physiol* 273:E99-107, 1997.

24. Pontzer, H, Durazo-Arvizu, R, Dugas, LR, Plange-Rhule, J, Bovet, P, Forrester, TE, Lambert, EV, Cooper, RS, Schoeller, DA, and Luke, A. Constrained total energy expenditure and metabolic adaptation to physical activity in adult humans. *Curr Biol* 26:410-417, 2016.

25. Robineau, J, Babault, N, Piscione, J, Lacome, M, and Bigard, AX. Specific training effects of concurrent aerobic and strength exercises depend on recovery duration. *J Strength Cond Res* 30:672-683, 2016.

26. Rossow, LM, Fukuda, DH, Fahs, CA, Loenneke, JP, and Stout, JR. Natural bodybuilding competition preparation and recovery: a 12-month case study. *Int J Sports Physiol Perform* 8:582-592, 2013.

27. Saris, WH and Schrauwen, P. Substrate oxidation differences between high- and low-intensity exercise are compensated over 24 hours in obese men. *Int J Obes Relat Metab Disord* 28:759-765, 2004.

28. Schoenfeld, BJ, Aragon, AA, Wilborn, CD, Krieger, JW, and Sonmez, GT. Body composition changes associated with fasted versus non-fasted aerobic exercise. *J Int Soc Sports Nutr* 11:54, 2014.

29. Schoenfeld, BJ, Contreras, B, Ogborn, D, Galpin, A, Krieger, J, and Sonmez, GT. Effects of varied versus constant loading zones on muscular adaptations in trained men. *Int J Sports Med* 37:442-447, 2016.

30. Schoenfeld, BJ, Ogborn, D, and Krieger, JW. Dose-response relationship between weekly resistance training volume and increases in muscle mass: a systematic review and meta-analysis. *J Sports Sci*:1-10, 2016.

31. Schoenfeld, BJ, Ogborn, D, and Krieger, JW. Effects of resistance training frequency on measures of muscle hypertrophy: a systematic review and meta-analysis. *Sports Med* 46:1689-1697, 2016.

32. Schoenfeld, BJ, Peterson, MD, Ogborn, D, Contreras, B, and Sonmez, GT. Effects of low- versus high-load resistance training on muscle strength and hypertrophy in well-trained men. *J Strength Cond Res* 29:2954-2963, 2015.

33. Schoenfeld, BJ, Pope, ZK, Benik, FM, Hester, GM, Sellers, J, Nooner, JL, Schnaiter, JA, Bond-Williams, KE, Carter, AS, Ross, CL, Just, BL, Henselmans, M, and Krieger, JW. Longer interset rest periods enhance muscle strength and hypertrophy in resistance-trained men. *J Strength Cond Res* 30:1805-1812, 2016.

34. Schoenfeld, BJ, Ratamess, NA, Peterson, MD, Contreras, B, Tiryaki-Sonmez, G, and Alvar, BA. Effects of different volume-equated resistance training loading strategies on muscular adaptations in well-trained men. *J Strength Cond Res* 28:2909-2918, 2014.

35. Schoenfeld, BJ, Vigotsky, A, Contreras, B, Golden, S, Alto, A, Larson, R, Winkelman, N, and Paoli, A. Differential effects of attentional focus strategies during long-term resistance training. *Eur J Sport Sci*:1-8, 2018.

36. Shepstone, TN, Tang, JE, Dallaire, S, Schuenke, MD, Staron, RS, and Phillips, SM. Short-term high- vs. low-velocity isokinetic lengthening training results in greater hypertrophy of the elbow flexors in young men. *J Appl Physiol (1985)* 98:1768-1776, 2005.

37. Simao, R, de Salles, BF, Figueiredo, T, Dias, I, and Willardson, JM. Exercise order in resistance training. *Sports Med* 42:251-265, 2012.

38. Snyder, BJ and Leech, JR. Voluntary increase in latissimus dorsi muscle activity during the lat pull-down following expert instruction. *J Strength Cond Res* 23:2204-2209, 2009.

39. Stults-Kolehmainen, MA, Bartholomew, JB, and Sinha, R. Chronic psychological stress impairs recovery of muscular function and somatic sensations over a 96-hour period. *J Strength Cond Res* 28:2007-2017, 2014.

40. Trexler, ET, Smith-Ryan, AE, and Norton, LE. Metabolic adaptation to weight loss: implications for the athlete. *J Int Soc Sports Nutr* 11:7, 2014.

41. Wernbom, M, Augustsson, J, and Thomee, R. The influence of frequency, intensity, volume, and mode of strength training on whole muscle cross-sectional area in humans. *Sports Med* 37:225-264, 2007.

42. West, DW and Phillips, SM. Associations of exercise-induced hormone profiles and gains in strength and hypertrophy in a large cohort after resistance training. *Eur J Appl Physiol* 112:2693-2702, 2012.

43. Willardson, JM. The application of training to failure in periodized multiple-set resistance exercise programs. *J Strength Cond Res* 21:628-631, 2007.

44. Wilson, JM, Marin, PJ, Rhea, MR, Wilson, SM, Loenneke, JP, and Anderson, JC. Concurrent training: a meta-analysis examining interference of aerobic and resistance exercise. *J Strength Cond Res* 26:2293-2307, 2011.

CHAPTER 10

1. Lote, C. *Principles of Renal Physiology*. 5th ed. New York: Springer, 12, 2012.

2. McBride, JJ, Guest, MM, and Scott, EL. The storage of the major liver components: emphasizing the relationship of glycogen to water in the liver and hydration of glycogen. *J Biol Chem* 139:943-952, 1941.

3. Olsson, KE and Saltin, B. Variation in total body water with muscle glycogen changes in man. *Acta Physiol Scand* 80:11-18, 1970.

4. Roedde, S, MacDougall, JD, Sutton, JR, and Green, HJ. Supercompensation of muscle glycogen in trained and untrained subjects. *Can J Appl Sport Sci* 11:42-46, 1986.

5. Toomey, CM, McCormack, WG, and Jakeman, P. The effect of hydration status on the measurement of lean tissue mass by dual-energy X-ray absorptiometry. *Eur J Appl Physiol* 117:567-574, 2017.

CHAPTER 12

1. Dulloo, AG, Jacquet, J, and Girardier, L. Poststarvation hyperphagia and body fat overshooting in humans: a role for feedback signals from lean and fat tissues. *Am J Clin Nutr* 65:717-723, 1997.

2. Dulloo, AG, Jacquet, J, and Montani, JP. How dieting makes some fatter: from a perspective of human body composition autoregulation. *Proc Nutr Soc* 71:379-389, 2012.

3. Garthe, I, Raastad, T, Refsnes, PE, and Sundgot-Borgen, J. Effect of nutritional intervention on body composition and performance in elite athletes. *Eur J Sport Sci* 13:295-303, 2013.

4. Halliday, TM, Loenneke, JP, and Davy, BM. Dietary intake, body composition, and menstrual cycle changes during competition preparation and recovery in a drug-free figure competitor: a case study. *Nutrients* 8:740, 2016.

5. Maclean, PS, Bergouignan, A, Cornier, MA, and Jackman, MR. Biology's response to dieting: the impetus for weight regain. *Am J Physiol Regul Integr Comp Physiol* 301:R581-600, 2011.

6. Rossow, LM, Fukuda, DH, Fahs, CA, Loenneke, JP, and Stout, JR. Natural bodybuilding competition preparation and recovery: a 12-month case study. *Int J Sports Physiol Perform* 8:582-592, 2013.

7. Trexler, ET, Hirsch, KR, Campbell, BI, and Smith-Ryan, AE. Physiological changes following competition in male and female physique athletes: a pilot study. *Int J Sport Nutr Exerc Metab* 27:458-466, 2017.

8. Trexler, ET, Smith-Ryan, AE, and Norton, LE. Metabolic adaptation to weight loss: implications for the athlete. *J Int Soc Sports Nutr* 11:7, 2014.

A

ab and thigh pose 114-115, 134-135, 158-159
age, and competition readiness 37
American Athletic Union (AAU) 3
American Natural Bodybuilding Federation (ANBF) 14
anabolic steroids 13
Arnold Classic competition 5
artificial sweeteners 64

B

back-load peaking protocol (glycogen supercompensation) 192-193
back-load peaking with cleanup day protocol 193-196
back or rear double biceps pose 110-111, 132-133, 156-157
back or rear lat spread pose 112-113
back pose 142-143, 164-165, 168-169
beginner class 31
beginners. See new competitors
bikini division 8, 28-29
    cutting water 187
    posing 95
    training program 82, 84-88
bingeing 209
blood volume maximum overload program 82, 83-84
bodybuilding division (men)
    about 16-17
    poses 96-121
    posing 93
bodybuilding division (women)
    about 22-23
    poses 96-121
    posing 93
body fat, monitoring 69, 209-210
body fat overshooting 209
body weight, monitoring 68-69, 210-212
British Amateur Weightlifting Association 2

C

caffeine 199
calcium deficiencies 9
caloric intake determination 52-54, 58
carbohydrate
    example needs for men 59
    example needs for women 62
    and peaking 183-185
    racial differences in need 58-59
    recommended intake 57-58
    sources 57
    sugar intake 57
    timing 65-66
cardio workouts
    amount 71-72
    in early 2000s 9
    fasted 72
    intensity of 72
    peak week 197
    timing with resistance training 73
cheat days 66
check-in 202
classic physique division
    about 7, 18-19
    poses 122-137
    posing 94
clenbuterol 13
collegiate class 32
competitors meeting 203
conditioning 33
contest preparation
    bikini division training program 82, 84-88
    blood volume maximum overload program 82, 83-84
    deloading 80
    energy expenditure, increasing 71-74
    hair removal 174

hair styling 176
jewelry 174
makeup 176
misinformed approaches to 8-9
multiple, within seasons 38, 207-208
overreaching 80
paperwork 176-177
posing music 173-174
posing practice 170-172, 173
posing suit 174
power block periodization program 81-82
range between contest seasons 38
resistance training 74-80
shoes 174
tanning 175
travel and hotel 177
contest readiness
    experienced competitors 37-38
    financial planning 40
    injury management 39
    mindset for 38-39
    new competitors 35-36
    optimal metabolic capacity 39
    plan adherence 39-40
    psychological readiness 41
contest selection and timing
    about 43
    appropriate rate of fat loss 44-45
    longer prep time benefits 45-46
    multiple, within seasons 38, 207-208
    prep time determination 43-44, 47-48
    selection factors 43-44
contest weekend
    after the show 205-206
    day before the show 202-203
    show day bag items 203
    show day logistics 203-205
    show day physique management 198-200
crab most muscular 118-119

D

dairy 9
Dark As 175
debut class 31
deloading 80
dextrins 183
Dianabol 3
diet breaks 46, 67
diuretics, prescription 13
Dream Tan 175
Drug Free Athletes Coalition (DFAC) 14
drug testing 202

E

energy balance 51-52
energy expenditure, increasing 71-74
enjoyment 214
ephedra 13
extracellular fluid 185

F

fat, dietary
    example needs for men 59
    example needs for women 62
    racial differences in need 58-59
    recommended intake 56
    sources 55-56
favorite classic pose 136-137
fiber intake 62-63
figure division
    about 8, 26-27
    poses 160-169
    posing 95
financial and expense planning 40
flat, definition 181

front double biceps pose 102-103, 128-129, 150-151
front lat spread pose 104-105
front-load peaking protocol 190
front pose 138-139, 160-161, 166-167
front standing relaxed pose 96-97, 122-123, 144-145
fruit 9
full, definition 181

G

genetics 37
glycogen storage 46, 65, 181, 184, 185
glycogen supercompensation peaking strategies 184-185, 192-193
Great Competition 2
grooming 202
growth hormones 13

H

hair removal 174, 202
hair styling 176, 202
hands clasped most muscular 120-121
hands on hips most muscular 116-117
hands overhead abdominal pose 114-115, 134-135, 158-159
history of bodybuilding
    early 1900s 2
    early physique competitions 1-2
    golden era 4
    late 20th century 4-5
    mid-20th century 3
    new divisions 7-8
holding water, definition 181
hunger 209

I

individuals with special needs 32
injuries, management for contest readiness 39
insulin 13
International Bodybuilding Association (IBA) 5
International Federation of Bodybuilding and Fitness (IFBB) 2, 3, 4, 7, 8, 12
International Natural Bodybuilding Association (INBA) 14
interstitial fluid 186-187
intracellular fluid 185

J

Jan Tana 175
jewelry 174
judging 204-205
junior class 31

L

lean, definition 181. See also stage-lean
leanness, achieving 45, 182
load look and peaking strategy choice 196

M

macronutrients 54-58
    baseline intake 180
    individual differences 58-62
Magazine of Physical Culture 1, 2
makeup 176
masters class 31
meal plans 60-61. See also nutrition
men's divisions
    choosing 30
    classes within 30-32
    classic physique 7, 18-19
    men's bodybuilding 16-17
    new divisions 7-8
    physique 7, 20-21
menstruation 208
metabolic adaptation 69
metabolic capacity 39
metabolic rate changes 208

mid-load peaking protocol 191
mind-muscle connection 76
mindset 38-39
mini cut 212
Mr. America competition 3
Mr. Olympia competition 2, 3, 4
Mr. Universe competition 2
Ms. Olympia competition 5
muscle glycogen 46, 65
muscle protein synthesis 64
muscle retention 45, 52
muscular definition 33
muscularity 33
muscular symmetry 33
music, posing 173-174

N
National Amateur Bodybuilding Association (NABBA) 3
National Gym Association (NGA) 5
National Physique Committee (NPC) 4, 7, 8, 12
new competitors
    attending a competition 36
    building a foundation 35-36
night show 205
nonexercise activity thermogenesis (NEAT) 73-74
North American Natural Bodybuilding Federation
        (NANBF) 14
novice class 31
nutrition
    bingeing 209
    caloric intake 52-54
    carbohydrate timing 65-66
    cheat days 66
    diet breaks 46, 67
    in early 2000s 9
    energy balance 51-52
    fiber 62-63
    hunger 209
    macronutrient differences, individual 58-62
    macronutrients 54-58
    meal frequency 64
    plateaus 69-70
    progress monitoring 68-69
    protein timing 64-65
    refeed days 46, 66-67
    vitamins and minerals 63-64

O
off-season 209-212
open class 31
Organization of Competitive Bodybuilders (OCB) 14
overreaching 80

P
peak week
    back-load peaking protocol 192-193
    back-load peaking with cleanup day protocol 193-196
    carbohydrates 183-185
    cardio during 197
    confusion about 179-180
    in early 2000s 9
    front-load peaking protocol 190
    glycogen supercompensation peaking strategies 192-193
    load look and strategy choice 196
    mid-load peaking protocol 191
    objective nonstarters 182-183
    objectives 181-182
    peaking network 189
    physique management peaking strategies 189-192
    prerequisites 180-181
    rapid back-load peaking protocol 195-196
    show day physique management 198-200
    slow back-load peaking protocol 191-192
    sodium-potassium balance 187-188

strategies 189-196
    terminology and definitions 181
    training plans 196-197
    water 185-187
performance-enhancing drugs
    drug testing 8
    and sanctions 11
    steroids 3, 4
physique division (men)
    about 7, 20-21
    poses 138-143
    posing 94
physique division (women)
    about 8, 24-25
    poses 144-159
    posing 94-95
physique management peaking strategies 189-192
poses
    bodybuilding division (men) 96-121
    bodybuilding division (women) 96-121
    classic physique division 122-137
    figure division 160-169
    physique division (men) 138-143
    physique division (women) 144-159
posing 91
    bikini (women) 95
    bodybuilding (men's and women's) 93
    classic physique (men) 94
    effective practice 170-172
    figure (women) 95
    music 173-174
    physique (men) 94
    physique (women) 94-95
    posing suit 174
    routines 170
    T-walks 170
postshow analysis 207
power block periodization program 81-82
prejudging 204-205
preparation time
    benefits of longer 45-46
    determination of 43-44, 47-48
professional class 32
Pro Tan 175
protein
    example needs for men 59
    example needs for women 62
    gender differences in need 58
    high-protein diets 56
    racial differences in need 58-59
    recommended intake 55
    sources 54
    timing 64-65, 66
psychological readiness 41, 212

R
rapid back-load peaking protocol 195-196
rate of fat loss 44-45, 47, 52, 53
rear standing relaxed pose 100-101, 126-127, 148-149
refeed days 46, 66-67
resistance training
    about 74-75
    exercise order 77
    exercise selection 75
    frequency 76, 77
    mind-muscle connection 76
    repetition range 77-78
    repetition tempo 78-79
    rest period length 78
    summary and additional factors 79-80
    training to failure 78
    volume 77
    workout length 79
ripped, definition 181

S
saccharides. *See* carbohydrate
salivary amylase 183
sanctions
    about 11
    drug-tested 12-14
    untested amateur 12
    untested professional 12
saunas 172
shoes 174
show day
    after the show 205-206
    day before the show 202-203
    logistics 203-205
    physique management 198-200
    show-day bag items 203
shredded, definition 181
side chest pose 106-107, 130-131
side chest with leg extended pose 152-153
side pose 140-141, 162-163
side standing relaxed pose 98-99, 124-125, 146-147
side triceps pose 108-109
side triceps with leg extended pose 154-155
skin, thinning 183
slow back-load peaking protocol 191-192
sodium-potassium balance 180, 181, 187-188
spilled (spilled over), definition 181
stage-lean 208-209
stage preparation 204
steroids 3, 5, 13
strength, monitoring 69
stress 46
strongman events 1
structural symmetry 33
submasters class 31
success and failure 213-214

T
tanning 175, 202
teen class 30
testosterone 13, 208
thyroid hormones 13
tight, definition 181
tracking nutrition 53-54
transformation class 32
travel and hotel 177

V
vascular, definition 181
vascularity 182, 199
vitamin D deficiencies 9
vitamins and minerals 63-64

W
water, peak week 180, 181, 183, 185-187
water retention 182
weightlifting 1, 2
women in bodybuilding
    caloric intake determination 58
    macronutrient needs 62
    menstruation abnormalities 208
    in mid-twentieth century 3
    Ms. Olympia competition 5
    21st-century changes 8
    weight fluctuations and menstruation 68
women's divisions
    bikini 8, 28-29
    bodybuilding 22-23
    choosing 30
    classes within 30-32
    figure 8, 26-27
    physique 8, 24-25
World Natural Bodybuilding Federation (WNBF) 5, 14
World Physique Alliance (WPA) 14

Peter J. Fitschen, PhD, CSCS, is the owner of FITbody and Physique, where he works full time as a contest prep coach. His combination of education and experience are unique in the sport of bodybuilding. He has a PhD in nutritional sciences from the University of Illinois, a master's degree in biology with a physiology concentration, and a bachelor's degree in biochemistry from the University of Wisconsin at La Crosse. As a researcher, Fitschen has coauthored 18 peer-reviewed publications, including several directly related to bodybuilding contest preparation. He is certified as a strength and conditioning specialist (CSCS) through the National Strength and Conditioning Association. He has been competing in natural bodybuilding since 2004 and won his natural pro card in 2012.

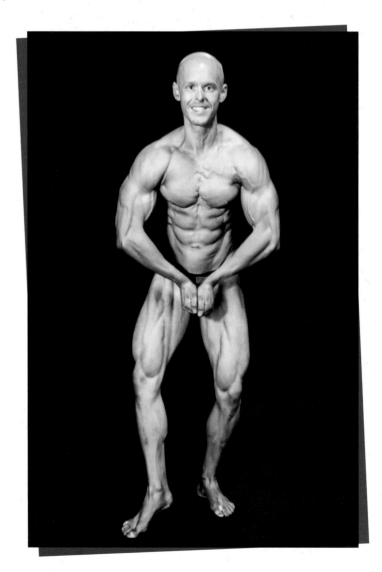

Cliff Wilson is a professional natural bodybuilder and one of the top physique coaches in the industry, having established himself through his work with competitive bodybuilders and powerlifters. Using a combination of scientifically proven methods and experience-driven techniques, Wilson's clients have amassed over 100 pro cards, more than 60 professional titles, and 9 world championships. His reputation as a coach has also allowed him to become a noted fitness author, with articles published in dozens of magazines and websites. Wilson is also a noted guest speaker who has given lectures around the world.

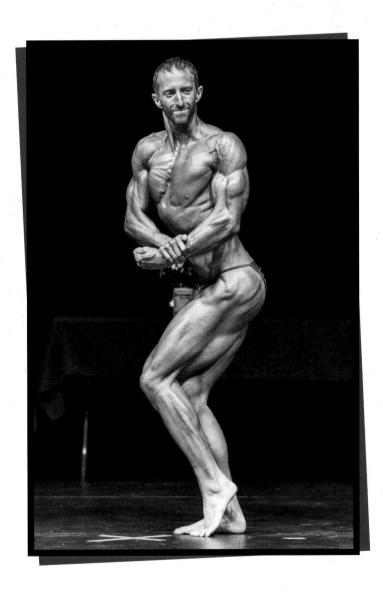

More Praise for *Bodybuilding*

"Having had years of experience in the area of bodybuilding competing, I know that nothing comes close to the detail and passion presented in this book by Cliff Wilson and Peter Fitschen. You need a winning team behind you, and here it is—the platinum standard to prep."

Torre Washington
Professional Bodybuilder and NASM-Certified Coach

"As a drug-free professional bodybuilding world champion, there are very few people I would trust to look over my contest prep; Cliff Wilson is one of those people. Cliff is a trailblazer in the contest prep arena, with his atypical yet scientifically valid and extremely effective methodologies. *Bodybuilding: The Complete Contest Preparation Handbook* takes a deep dive into these methodologies, thoroughly discussing the basics and the intricacies of all aspects of a proper contest preparation. Whether you are a newbie or a veteran competitor, this book is a must-read."

Doug Miller
President and CEO of Core Nutritionals LLC

"If you are looking for a comprehensive and thorough manual on physique competitions, look no further! From the attention to fine detail on what helps a competitor perfect their physique to special considerations on the psychological aspects of competing, this book has upmost value to any competitor, whether you are a beginner or a pro. As a dietitian, I was highly impressed with the attention to detail in both training and nutritional recommendations that followed an evidence-based approach for optimizing health during a contest prep. I highly recommend this resource to anyone who competes or wants to learn more about dieting to enhance their physique."

Lacey Dunn, RD, LD, CPT

"Having been in the contest prep industry for many years as a coach and competitor, I often forget the types of questions first-time competitors may have. I would recommend this comprehensive guide to anyone interested in competing."

Adam Atkinson
Contest Prep Coach for See You Later Leaner

"As a long-time competitor, bodybuilding pro, and contest prep coach, I can say this is without a doubt the most up-to-date and extensive reference for information on the bodybuilding preparation process that I've ever come across. Cliff and Pete have really put together something special here, with a great wealth of knowledge and immaculate attention to detail, all backed up by modern science and research."

Corbin Pierson
Professional Bodybuilder

"Whenever people ask me for motivation or express doubt, I tell them, 'your body is capable of achieving far more than you think.' With the help of Peter and Cliff's book, you will be amazed at your results."

Maurice Benton
IFBB Pro

"*Bodybuilding: The Complete Contest Preparation Handbook* is a breath of fresh air in an industry filled with outdated and misguided information. Cliff and Peter have taken their years of research experience and time spent in the trenches to bring you a blend of scientific principles of competition prep with the delicate art of coaching that is required to bring your best look possible."

Austin Current, BSc, CSCS
IFBB Pro, Educator, and Physique Coach

"Bodybuilding is a noninstitutionalized sport that you can't learn in high school or a team organization. This book encompasses that practical foundation that bodybuilders usually have to frustratingly learn on their own. Whether you are starting your first prep or looking for the fine details that a professional needs, this book covers it all with an easy-to-read, evidence-based approach."

Ryan Dorris
Pro Natural Bodybuilder

"*Bodybuilding* is a highly comprehensive book that covers every single aspect of competition prep. From off-season to prep to show day to post show, Cliff and Peter dive deep into it all, blending both an evidence-based approach and their own practical coaching experience. The book is written in easy-to-understand language while still providing full citations for all the applicable science in the field."

Laurin Conlin, MS
IFBB Bikini Pro and Research Associate at USF Physique Enhancement Laboratory

"This is easily the most comprehensive book on contest preparation I have ever seen. I've been coaching for 12 years, and not only did I pick up new tools for my toolbox, but it was great to review some things I may have forgotten. I recommend this to anyone at any level of bodybuilding."

Jason M. Theobald, AFPA
Owner of Scooby Prep and Co-owner of Nuethix Formulations

"*Bodybuilding: The Complete Contest Preparation Handbook* is really what the title claims it is . . . COMPLETE. Being in this industry as a full-time coach, promoter, judge, and natural pro bodybuilder for over five years, I have not seen a book that covers the sport in this much detail. This is a MUST-HAVE for anyone looking to compete—especially the novice competitor or someone looking to learn more about the sport!"

Matt Jackson
Owner of MEAT (Make Everyday A Transformation) and IPE Pro Masters Bodybuilder

"If you're new to bodybuilding or a seasoned veteran, this book is for you! It gives you anything and everything you need to know about competing and the mind-set involved with it!"

Mike Pucci
Pro Natural Bodybuilder and Online Coach at Team Unique Prep

"Always work to find that middle ground, and never forget that we are not defined by the way we look on show day; it is merely a snapshot of our lives as competitors. In *Bodybuilding*, Cliff helps you understand every aspect of the process and every look that comes with it."

Samaiyah Council
Pro Women's Physique Hybrid Athlete

"If you're a first-time competitor or a veteran to the sport, it will not matter—everyone can learn from this book. And, if you want to get ahead of the game, then I suggest *Bodybuilding: The Complete Preparation Handbook*. Learn the right way of bodybuilding and learn how to approach it by responding to what your body does naturally."

Ty Young
NPC Competitor and Coach

"Nobody knows the art of bodybuilding and competition prep quite like Cliff Wilson and Peter Fitschen. Their many years of experience and evidence-based methods have produced exceptional results, and this book is bursting with quality information every coach and competitor should know. Whether you're looking to step up your physique or take your coaching to the next level, this book is a must-read."

Anna McManamey
WBFF Bikini Pro and Competition Prep Coach

"*Bodybuilding: The Complete Contest Preparation Handbook* is truly an invaluable tool for both bodybuilding coaches and athletes alike. It provides a comprehensive and up-to-date look at both the evidence and practice of bodybuilding as a whole, delving into each particular phase of a contest prep. This book will give anybody who is reading it a complete basis and understanding of the all of the major components that make up a successful prep and a successful bodybuilder. I recommend it without hesitation."

Leanna Carr
Natural Figure Pro and Performance and Fitness Coach

"I can say that without a doubt Cliff is one of the most well respected and knowledgeable coaches within the bodybuilding industry today. Cliff's success is obviously not by accident, as he possesses the perfect mix of passion, knowledge, experience, and an undeniable competitor's edge, which is what makes his resume so impressive. In the fitness industry, to find someone who is so successful yet so humble is rare, and this is by far one of my favorite parts about Cliff!"

Sal Frisella
President of 1st Phorm

"Peter Fitschen and Cliff Wilson provide us with the most comprehensive handbook for competitive physique athletes out there. This book is a potent ally for athletes and coaches alike who want to maximize their contest preparation."

Valentin Tambosi
Prep Coach and Pro Natural Bodybuilder

You read the book—now complete an exam to earn continuing education credit!

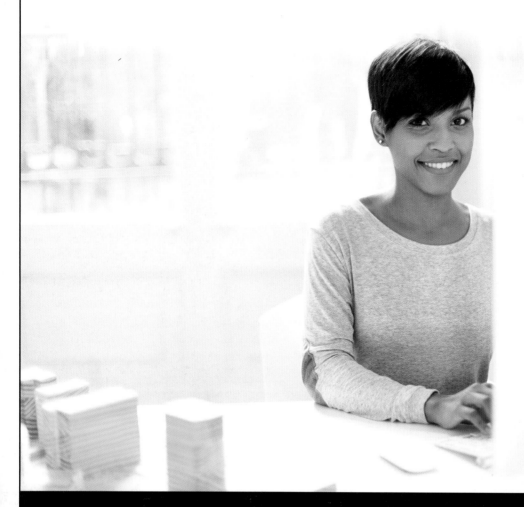

Congratulations on successfully preparing for this continuing education exam!

If you would like to earn CE credit, please visit

www.HumanKinetics.com/CE-Exam-Access

for complete instructions on how to access your exam. Take advantage of a discounted rate by entering promo code **BB2020** when prompted.

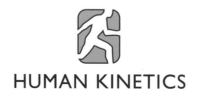

HUMAN KINETICS